PET in the Management of Hematologic Malignancies

Editors

ABASS ALAVI
LALE KOSTAKOGLU
GARY A. ULANER
JAKUB SVOBODA

PET CLINICS

www.pet.theclinics.com

Consulting Editor
ABASS ALAVI

July 2019 • Volume 14 • Number 3

ELSEVIER

1600 John F. Kennedy Boulevard • Suite 1800 • Philadelphia, Pennsylvania, 19103-2899

http://www.pet.theclinics.com

PET CLINICS Volume 14, Number 3
July 2019 ISSN 1556-8598, ISBN-13: 978-0-323-67878-0

Editor: John Vassallo (j.vassallo@elsevier.com)
Developmental Editor: Casey Potter

PET Clinics (ISSN 1556-8598) is published quarterly by Elsevier Inc., 360 Park Avenue South, New York, NY 10010-1710. Months of issue are January, April, July, and October. Periodicals postage paid at New York, NY, and additional mailing offices. Subscription prices per year are $240.00 (US individuals), $396.00 (US institutions), $100.00 (US students), $279.00 (Canadian individuals), $446.00 (Canadian institutions), $140.00 (Canadian students), $275.00 (foreign individuals), $446.00 (foreign institutions), and $140.00 (foreign students). To receive student and resident rate, orders must be accompanied by name of affiliated institution, date of term, and the signature of program/residency coordinator on institution letterhead. Orders will be billed at individual rate until proof of status is received. Foreign air speed delivery is included in all Clinics subscription prices. All prices are subject to change without notice. POSTMASTER: Send address changes to PET Clinics, Elsevier Health Sciences Division, Subscription Customer Service, 3251 Riverport Lane, Maryland Heights, MO 63043. **Customer Service: 1-800-654-2452 (U.S. and Canada); 314-447-8871 (outside U.S. and Canada). Fax: 314-447-8029. E-mail: journalscustomerservice-usa@elsevier.com (for print support); journalsonlinesupport-usa@elsevier.com (for online support).**

Reprints. For copies of 100 or more of articles in this publication, please contact the Commercial Reprints Department, Elsevier Inc., 360 Park Avenue South, New York, NY 10010-1710. Tel.: 212-633-3874; Fax: 212-633-3820; E-mail: reprints@elsevier.com.

PET Clinics is covered in MEDLINE/PubMed (Index Medicus).

Contributors

CONSULTING EDITOR

ABASS ALAVI, MD, MD (Hon), PhD (Hon), DSc (Hon)
Professor of Radiology, Division of Nuclear Medicine, Department of Radiology, Hospital of the University of Pennsylvania, University of Pennsylvania Perelman School of Medicine, Philadelphia, Pennsylvania, USA

EDITORS

ABASS ALAVI, MD, MD (Hon), PhD (Hon), DSc (Hon)
Professor of Radiology, Division of Nuclear Medicine, Department of Radiology, Hospital of the University of Pennsylvania, University of Pennsylvania Perelman School of Medicine, Philadelphia, Pennsylvania, USA

LALE KOSTAKOGLU, MD, MPH
Professor of Radiology, Chief, Nuclear Medicine and Molecular Imaging, Department of Radiology, Icahn School of Medicine at Mount Sinai, New York, New York, USA

GARY A. ULANER, MD, PhD
Memorial Sloan Kettering Cancer Center, New York, New York, USA

JAKUB SVOBODA, MD
Division of Hematology Oncology, Perelman Center for Advanced Medicine, Lymphoma Program, Abramson Cancer Center, University of Pennsylvania, Philadelphia, Pennsylvania, USA

AUTHORS

ABASS ALAVI, MD, MD (Hon), PhD (Hon), DSc (Hon)
Professor of Radiology, Division of Nuclear Medicine, Department of Radiology, Hospital of the University of Pennsylvania, University of Pennsylvania Perelman School of Medicine, Philadelphia, Pennsylvania, USA

CYRUS AYUBCHA, BA
Department of Radiology, University of Pennsylvania, Philadelphia, Pennsylvania, USA

STEVEN M. BAIR, MD
Lymphoma Program, Abramson Cancer Center, University of Pennsylvania, Philadelphia, Pennsylvania, USA

BART BARLOGIE, MD
Director of Myeloma Research, Mount Sinai Hospital/Tisch Cancer Institute, New York, New York, USA

MERAL BEKSAC, MD
Professor, Department of Hematology, Ankara University School of Medicine, Ankara, Turkey

STEPHEN M. BROSKI, MD
Department of Radiology, Mayo Clinic,
Rochester, Minnesota, USA

STÉPHANE CHAUVIE, PhD
Chief, Department of Medical Physics, 'Santa
Croce e Carle' Hospital, Cuneo, Italy

KATRINA N. GLAZEBROOK, MD
Department of Radiology, Mayo Clinic,
Rochester, Minnesota, USA

LALE KOSTAKOGLU, MD, MPH
Professor of Radiology, Chief, Nuclear
Medicine and Molecular Imaging,
Department of Radiology, Icahn School of
Medicine at Mount Sinai, New York, New York,
USA

ESHA KOTHEKAR, MD
Department of Radiology, University of
Pennsylvania, Philadelphia, Pennsylvania,
USA

SHAJI KUMAR, MD
Professor of Medicine, Division of
Hematology, Mayo Clinic, Rochester,
Minnesota, USA

DEEPU MADDURI, MD
Assistant Professor, Mount Sinai Hospital/
Tisch Cancer Institute, New York, New York,
USA

ANTHONY R. MATO, MD, MSCE
CLL Program, Leukemia Service, Division of
Hematological Oncology, Memorial Sloan
Kettering Cancer Center, New York, New York,
USA

CRISTINA NANNI, MD
Metropolitan nuclear medicine, Azienda
Ospedaliera-Universitaria di Bologna S. Orsola
Malpighi, Bologna, Italy

GRZEGORZ S. NOWAKOWSKI, MD
Division of Hematology, Mayo Clinic,
Rochester, Minnesota, USA

ELGIN OZKAN, MD
Assistant Professor, Department of Nuclear
Medicine, Ankara University School of
Medicine, Ankara, Turkey

WILLIAM Y. RAYNOR, BS
Department of Radiology, University of
Pennsylvania, Drexel University College of
Medicine, Philadelphia, Pennsylvania, USA

JOANNA M. RHODES, MD
Division of Hematology and Oncology,
Department of Medicine, Hospital of the
University of Pennsylvania, Philadelphia,
Pennsylvania, USA

SIAVASH MEHDIZADEH SERAJ, MD, MHM
Department of Radiology, University of
Pennsylvania, Philadelphia, Pennsylvania, USA

GULDANE CENGIZ SEVAL, MD
Department of Hematology, Ankara University
School of Medicine, Ankara, Turkey

JAKUB SVOBODA, MD
Division of Hematology Oncology, Perelman
Center for Advanced Medicine, Lymphoma
Program, Abramson Cancer Center, University
of Pennsylvania, Philadelphia, Pennsylvania,
USA

THOMAS WERNER, MSc
Department of Radiology, University of
Pennsylvania, Philadelphia, Pennsylvania, USA

DANI P. YELLANKI, BS
Department of Radiology, University of
Pennsylvania, Philadelphia, Pennsylvania, USA

MAHDI ZIRAKCHIAN ZADEH, MD, MHM
Department of Radiology, University of
Pennsylvania, Department of Radiology,
Children's Hospital of Philadelphia,
Philadelphia, Pennsylvania, USA

ELENA ZAMAGNI, MD, PhD
"Seràgnoli" Institute of Hematology, Bologna
University School of Medicine, Bologna, Italy

Contents

PET imaging with fluorodeoxyglucose (FDG), integrated with PET/computed tomography (FDG-PET/CT), is an effective management tool of diffuse large B-cell lymphoma (DLBCL). The results of end-of-treatment (EOT) FDG-PET/CT are more accurate for detection of active disease with residual masses on CT. Complete response defined by EOT FDG-PET/CT (PET-CR) correlates with long-term outcome of patients. Treatment efficacy is determined using EOT PET/CT rather than progression-free survival (PFS) for clinical trials assessing novel drugs. If the correlation of EOT PET/CT with PFS is further proven in large studies and meta-analyses, EOT PET-CR could serve as an expedited novel endpoint replacing PFS.

Lymphoma is a potentially curable disease; however, the clinical challenge lies in further improvement of outcomes. PET with fludeoxyglucose is an effective imaging tool. PET-derived quantitative metrics have raised significant interest to be used as a prognostic factor to complement clinical parameters for treatment decisions. The most optimized use of these quantitative PET metrics, however, will be possible with the standardization of imaging procedures. In this article, we review the technical and methodological considerations related to PET-derived quantitative metrics, and the relevant published data to emphasize the potential value of these metrics in patient prognosis and treatment response in lymphoma.

The role of ^{18}F-fluorodeoxyglucose PET/computed tomography in hematological malignancies continues to expand in disease diagnosis, staging, and management. A key advantage of PET over other imaging modalities is its ability to quantify tracer uptake, which can be used to determine degree of disease activity. Although tracer uptake with PET is conventionally measured in focal lesions, novel quantitative techniques are being investigated that set objective protocols and produce robust parameters that represent total disease activity portrayed by PET. This article discusses recent advances in PET quantification that can improve reliability and accuracy of characterizing hematological malignancies.

Consistencies between independent studies confirm the negative prognostic value of extramedullary disease and greater than 3 focal lesions, whereas the role of standardized uptake value is more conflicting. Standardization of the technique is ongoing.

Fludeoxyglucose F 18 PET/Computed Tomography Evaluation of Therapeutic Response in Multiple Myeloma

Shaji Kumar, Katrina N. Glazebrook, and Stephen M. Broski

Multiple myeloma is a malignancy of terminally differentiated plasma cells representing the second most common hematological malignancy. The recognition that disease outside the marrow can significantly influence the outcome of patients has highlighted the importance of imaging to define presence of tumor. Recent studies have demonstrated an added value of using imaging to assess presence of disease both inside and outside the marrow. To this end, the response criteria have been revised to include PET/computed tomography to be used in conjunction with bone marrow assessment to determine minimal residual disease status.

PET/Computed Tomography in Chronic Lymphocytic Leukemia and Richter Transformation

Joanna M. Rhodes and Anthony R. Mato

Chronic lymphocytic leukemia (CLL) is the most common leukemia in the United States. In 1-10% of cases, it can undergo Richter's transformation (RT) to either diffuse large B cell lymphoma (DLBCL) or Hodgkin's lymphoma (HL). Diagnosis requires histologic confirmation by tissue biopsy. PET/CT has been studied to in several series to look at its predictive value for identifying RT in biopsies. in this review, we will discuss the role of PET/CT to identify RT in patients CLL and its utility in clinical practice.

PET-Computed Tomography in Myeloma: Current Overview and Future Directions

Deepu Madduri and Bart Barlogie

The treatment landscape of multiple myeloma (MM) has been rapidly evolving, leading to improved survival for patients. Given the existence of effective treatment strategies, it is important to not only have better response criteria but also have imaging modalities capable of measuring treatment response, because most patients present with focal bone marrow/bone lesions not captured by myeloma protein and bone marrow examination. Whole body skeletal survey has been considered as a "gold standard" for the determination of the extent of myeloma bone disease at diagnosis.

PET CLINICS

SERIES OF RELATED INTEREST

MRI Clinics of North America
Available at: MRI.theclinics.com
Neuroimaging Clinics of North America
Available at: Neuroimaging.theclinics.com
Radiologic Clinics of North America
Available at: Radiologic.theclinics.com

THE CLINICS ARE AVAILABLE ONLINE!
Access your subscription at:
www.theclinics.com

PROGRAM OBJECTIVE

The goal of the *PET Clinics* is to keep practicing radiologists and radiology residents up to date with current clinical practice in positron emission tomography by providing timely articles reviewing the state of the art in patient care.

TARGET AUDIENCE

Practicing radiologists, radiology residents, and other health care professionals who provide patient care utilizing radiologic findings.

LEARNING OBJECTIVES

Upon completion of this activity, participants will be able to:

1. Review PET as a valuable prognostic tool for hematologic malignancies
2. Discuss new concepts for PET-based evaluation of patients with multiple myeloma
3. Recognize PET/CT as a staging and evaluation imaging tool, as well as a predictor of prognosis in multiple myeloma

ACCREDITATION

The Elsevier Office of Continuing Medical Education (EOCME) is accredited by the Accreditation Council for Continuing Medical Education (ACCME) to provide continuing medical education for physicians.

The EOCME designates this enduring material for a maximum of 15 *AMA PRA Category 1 Credit*(s)™. Physicians should claim only the credit commensurate with the extent of their participation in the activity.

All other health care professionals requesting continuing education credit for this enduring material will be issued a certificate of participation.

DISCLOSURE OF CONFLICTS OF INTEREST

The EOCME assesses conflict of interest with its instructors, faculty, planners, and other individuals who are in a position to control the content of CME activities. All relevant conflicts of interest that are identified are thoroughly vetted by EOCME for fair balance, scientific objectivity, and patient care recommendations. EOCME is committed to providing its learners with CME activities that promote improvements or quality in healthcare and not a specific proprietary business or a commercial interest.

The planning committee, staff, authors and editors listed below have identified no financial relationships or relationships to products or devices they or their spouse/life partner have with commercial interest related to the content of this CME activity:

Abass Alavi, MD, MD(Hon), PhD(Hon), DSc(Hon); Cyrus Ayubcha, BA; Steven M. Bair, MD; Bart Barlogie, MD; Meral Beksac, MD; Stephen M. Broski, MD; Stéphane Chauvie, PhD; Katrina N. Glazebrook, MD; Alison Kemp; Lale Kostakoglu, MD, MPH; Esha Kothekar, MD; Deepu Madduri, MD; Cristina Nanni, MD; Grzegorz S. Nowakowski, MD; Elgin Ozkan, MD; William Y. Raynor, BS; Joanna M. Rhodes, MD; Siavash Mehdizadeh Seraj, MD; Guldane Cengiz Seval, MD; John Vassallo; Vignesh Viswanathan; Thomas Werner, MSE; Dani P. Yellanki, BA; Mahdi Zirakchian Zadeh, MD, MHM.

The planning committee, staff, authors and editors listed below have identified financial relationships or relationships to products or devices they or their spouse/life partner have with commercial interest related to the content of this CME activity:

Shaji Kumar, MD: is a consultant/advisor for and receives research support from AbbVie, Inc, Celgene Corporation, Janssen Global Services, LLC, Merck Sharp & Dohme Corp., Novartis AG, F. Hoffmann-La Roche Ltd, sanofi-aventis U.S. LLC, Takeda Pharmaceutical Company Limited, Kite Pharma, Inc., and AstraZeneca; is a consultant/advisor for Adaptive Biotechnologies and Oncopeptides AB.

Anthony R. Mato, MD, MSCE: is a consultant/advisor for DAVA Oncology and Pharmacyclics LLC, is a consultant/advisor for and receives research support from AbbVie Inc., Acerta Pharma, Celgene Corporation, Janssen Global Services, LLC, Sunesis Pharmaceuticals, Inc, and TG Therapeutics, Inc.

Jakub Svoboda, MD: is a consultant/advisor for Kite Pharma and Kyowa Kirin Pharmaceutical Development, Inc., receives research support from Merck Sharp & Dohme Corp., Regeneron, and TG Therapeutics, Inc., and is a consultant/advisor and receives research support from Bristol-Myers Squibb Company, Pharmacyclics LLC, and Seattle Genetics, Inc.

UNAPPROVED/OFF-LABEL USE DISCLOSURE

The EOCME requires CME faculty to disclose to the participants:

1. When products or procedures being discussed are off-label, unlabelled, experimental, and/or investigational (not US Food and Drug Administration [FDA] approved); and
2. Any limitations on the information presented, such as data that are preliminary or that represent ongoing research, interim analyses, and/or unsupported opinions. Faculty may discuss information about pharmaceutical agents that is outside of FDA-approved labelling. This information is intended solely for CME and is not intended to promote off-label use of these medications. If you have any questions, contact the medical affairs department of the manufacturer for the most recent prescribing information.

TO ENROLL

To enroll in the *PET Clinics* Continuing Medical Education program, call customer service at 1-800-654-2452 or sign up online at http://www.theclinics.com/home/cme. The CME program is available to subscribers for an additional annual fee of USD $235.

METHOD OF PARTICIPATION

In order to claim credit, participants must complete the following:

1. Complete enrolment as indicated above.
2. Read the activity.
3. Complete the CME Test and Evaluation. Participants must achieve a score of 70% on the test. All CME Tests and Evaluations must be completed online.

CME INQUIRIES/SPECIAL NEEDS

For all CME inquiries or special needs, please contact elsevierCME@elsevier.com

Preface

Evolving Role of PET Imaging in Hematologic Malignancies

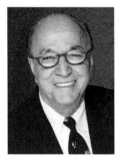

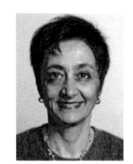

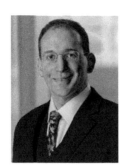

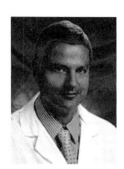

Abass Alavi, MD   Lale Kostakoglu, MD, MPH   Gary A. Ulaner, MD, PhD   Jakub Svoboda, MD

Editors

The introduction of fludeoxyglucose (FDG)-PET to the medical imaging arena has had a major impact on the evolution of radiologic techniques for assessing various diseases and disorders over the past four decades. The original intent of investigators at the University of Pennsylvania was to determine the role of FDG in evaluating brain function in normal aging and neuropsychiatric disorders. However, soon after these initial studies investigating central nervous system maladies, FDG was employed to determine the degree of aggressiveness of brain tumors. Soon after the introduction of PET-based body imaging instruments, this compound was found to be of great value in diagnosing, staging, monitoring response to treatment, and detecting the recurrence of a multitude of malignant disorders. This trend has continued over the past decades as the essential role of FDG-PET scanning as a powerful imaging modality has been proven and well established in the practice of medical, surgical, and radiation oncology. By now, the imaging community has realized that, without applications of FDG in solid tumors, PET imaging would have never survived.

In the past two decades, PET has been shown to play a major role in assessing hematologic malignancies. Initially, PET was utilized to stage patients with lymphomas and demonstrated its superiority over conventional radiologic techniques, such as computed tomography (CT), by monitoring response and detecting recurrence

because of its high sensitivity and specificity. However, the role of this very powerful modality has not been adequately assessed in other hematologic malignancies, such as multiple myeloma and leukemias. By now, it is clear that FDG and other powerful PET tracers are able to demonstrate the extent of the disease within and outside bone marrow, determine the degree of aggressiveness of the involved sites, and assess the efficacy of various therapeutic interventions. Therefore, it is very timely for the molecular community to realize that PET imaging has an essential place in this discipline similar to that of solid tumors for managing these relatively common malignancies.

In this issue of *PET Clinics*, we have described the latest developments in the usefulness of PET in all domains related to hematologic malignancies and how it can play a major role as an imaging modality in optimal management of these potentially fatal cancers. In particular, we have emphasized the importance of novel quantitative techniques that are not provided by other imaging modalities, such as CT or MR imaging. These include global disease assessment by advanced analysis schemes, which allow measurement of total burden of disease in the bone marrow and in the extramedullary sites that are known to be involved in these malignancies. Also, we have discussed the development of some other novel tracers, including sodium fluoride (NaF), for assessing

PET Clin 14 (2019) xi–xii
https://doi.org/10.1016/j.cpet.2019.03.011
1556-8598/19/© 2019 Published by Elsevier Inc.

multiple myeloma and other destructive malignancies. NaF-PET imaging will play a critical role in detecting fractures due to osteoporosis following diffuse spread of the disease in the skeleton. Therefore, this issue will be of great value to the oncologists who are actively involved in managing patients with these cancers.

Abass Alavi, MD
Department of Radiology
Hospital of the University of Pennsylvania
3400 Spruce Street
Philadelphia, PA 19104, USA

Lale Kostakoglu, MD, MPH
Icahn School of Medicine at Mount Sinai
1190 Fifth Avenue
New York, NY 10029, USA

Gary A. Ulaner, MD, PhD
Memorial Sloan Kettering Cancer Center
1275 York Avenue
Box 77
New York, NY 10065, USA

Jakub Svoboda, MD
Division of Hematology Oncology
Perelman Center for Advanced Medicine
12th Floor, South Pavilion
Office #12-158
3400 Civic Center Boulevard
Philadelphia, PA 19104, USA

E-mail addresses:
Abass.Alavi@uphs.upenn.edu (A. Alavi)
lale.kostakoglu@mountsinai.org (L. Kostakoglu)
ulanerg@mskcc.org (G.A. Ulaner)
Jakub.Svoboda@uphs.upenn.edu (J. Svoboda)

End-of-Treatment PET/ Computed Tomography Response in Diffuse Large B-Cell Lymphoma

Lale Kostakoglu, MD, MPH[a],*,
Grzegorz S. Nowakowski, MD[b]

KEYWORDS

- FDG-PET/CT ● Diffuse large B- cell lymphoma ● End-of-treatment PET-CT ● Prediction of outcome

KEY POINTS

- To improve the objectivity in interpretation of FDG PET/CT imaging and determine prognosis at baseline in lymphoma, the PET-based quantitative parameters including volumetric measurements have been under investigation.
- Quantitative PET assessment with MTV and TLG seems to be a highly promising method to predict outcome of lymphoma patients.
- However, this methodology is still in an evolutionary phase and, there is no consensus regarding the optimal segmentation algorithm or the quantitative index to assess the actual metabolic disease burden.
- Further trials investigating the prognostic and predictive values of MTV are warranted in large, standardized, prospective data sets for both the internal and external validation of this method to prove or refute a role to improve on the prognostic value of conventional risk stratifying systems in lymphoma.

INTRODUCTION

Diffuse large B-cell lymphoma (DLBCL) is a highly heterogeneous disease with clinicopathologic and genotypic diversity. The combination of anti-CD20 antibody, rituximab, with conventional chemotherapy that consists of cyclophosphamide, doxorubicin, vincristine, and prednisone (RCHOP) significantly improved survival. Nonetheless, approximately 40% of patients will relapse after first-line therapy and only a fraction of these patients will be cured.[1]

In oncology drug development, most phase II-III clinical trials evaluate whether a drug provides a survival benefit to the patient. In the United States,

the regulatory agency, the Food and Drug Administration (FDA), may also permit accelerated approval of a drug based on an earlier clinical endpoint that is reasonably likely to predict an effect on morbidity or mortality.[2] After the approval, if the drug profile fails to demonstrate the expected clinical benefit, the FDA may withdraw approval of the drug.

Progression-free survival (PFS) is a traditionally used and preferred surrogate endpoint for frontline lymphoma trials to measure treatment effects. This is because in patients with DLBCL, the maintenance of a progression-free status for a minimum of 2 years after the first-line treatment is one of the strongest predictors of long-term

[a] Department of Radiology, Icahn School of Medicine at Mount Sinai, New York, NY 10029, USA; [b] Division of Hematology, Mayo Clinic, 200 First Street Southwest, Rochester, MN 55901, USA
* Corresponding author. Department of Radiology, Icahn School of Medicine at Mount Sinai, One Gustave Levy Place, Box 1141, New York, NY 10022.
E-mail addresses: lale.kostakoglu@mssm.edu; lale.kostakoglu@mountsinai.org

PET Clin 14 (2019) 307–315
https://doi.org/10.1016/j.cpet.2019.03.001

survival.[3] Most patients whose disease relapses within the first 2 years of first-line treatment have a significantly inferior survival even with salvage therapies compared with those who are progression-free for more than 2 years after treatment. In this context, the clinical dilemma is that at least 2 years should elapse to reach the median PFS to determine treatment efficacy. This long observation period of at least 2 years brings inefficiency from both the patients and the health economics point of view. Therefore, a faster predictive endpoint that could be used as a surrogate for long-term outcome is an unmet medical need to minimize unwarranted side effects and reduce the cost of a potentially ineffective drug. Perhaps equally importantly, end-of-treatment (EOT) PET surrogacy for outcome would allow implementation of early stopping rules in front-line phase 3 trials. Currently, it remains impractical to suspend the trials for interim efficacy analysis based on PFS due to the long follow-up time required. Utilization of EOT PET–complete response (CR) rates in early efficacy analysis would allow minimization of patients' exposure to potentially ineffective therapy while allowing early shifting of development and resources to more promising combinations.

The 18-fluorodeoxyglucose positron emission tomography (FDG–PET) with computed tomography (PET/CT) has been incorporated into the standard assessment of DLBCL, after the publication of the Revised Response Criteria for Malignant Lymphoma[4] and, more recently, with the widespread application of Lugano guidelines.[5,6] The latest Lugano response guidelines incorporated the Deauville 5-point scale (D 5PS) as an assessment tool for FDG-PET/CT interpretation, providing a clear definition of response status using a categorical scale. PET/CT imaging has proved to be an effective diagnostic tool in determining extent of disease in DLBCL leading to a change in stage of disease in up to 20% to 40% of patients, and leads to a change in the treatment in 5% to 15%.[7–13] A CR based on EOT PET/CT, that is, PET-CR, can be used as a surrogate of outcome, which affords a significantly earlier measurement of treatment effect than PFS. The presence of an EOT FDG-avid mass, non–PET-CR, in such cases also helps determine the need for consolidation radiation.

PET–COMPLETE RESPONSE AS A PREDICTOR OF OUTCOME IN PATIENTS WITH DIFFUSE LARGE B-CELL LYMPHOMA

Although the role of the midtreatment imaging with PET/CT scan is controversial, multiple studies,

including meta-analyses, have reported a strong correlation between EOT PET-CR and clinical outcome as measured by PFS, event-free survival (EFS), and/or overall survival (OS) in patients with DLBCL after standard first-line chemoimmunotherapy[14–29] (Table 1).

In a meta-analysis, Zhu and colleagues[14] investigated the impact of PET-CR on progression and survival in 13 selected studies in 1160 patients with B-cell non-Hodgkin lymphoma (NHL) treated with rituximab-containing chemotherapy. This study confirmed the independent prognostic value of PET-CR in patients with DLBCL treated with first-line R-chemotherapy without statistical heterogeneity. The combined hazard ratios (HRs) of EOT PET for PFS and OS in DLBCL were 6.75 (95% confidence interval [CI] 1.72–26.5) and 5.91 (95% CI 3.15–11.09), respectively, although the corresponding HRs for interim PET for PFS and OS in DLBCL were inferior at 4.4 ($P = .11$) and 3.99 ($P = .46$), respectively.[14]

Prospective Studies Supporting a Role for Surrogacy for PET–Complete Response

Most prospective studies reporting on the predictive value of EOT PET-CR primarily investigated the interim PET as an early predictor of response and outcome.[15–20] Although the EOT PET results were analyzed as a comparator to the results of interim PET, collectively, these studies confirmed the high predictive value of EOT PET-CR and almost all suggested that interim PET/CT was inferior to EOT PET/CT as a predictor of outcome, therefore it would be an inappropriate tool for designing risk-adaptive therapy in chemotherapy-naïve patients with DLBCL.

In an earlier prospective study conducted in 50 patients with advanced-stage DLBCL who were treated with standard RCHOP chemotherapy, Cashen and colleagues[15] demonstrated that EOT FDG-PET/CT had a high positive predictive value and negative predictive value (NPV) (71% and 80%, respectively) and was significantly associated with PFS and OS ($P<.001$). PET scans were interpreted using International Harmonization Project (IHP) criteria.[4,30] Not surprisingly, interim PET performed during treatment was poorly associated with OS. EOT PET imaging had a high positive (71%) and negative (80%) predictive value for relapse or progression with a median follow-up of 33.9 months. The weaknesses of our study were that baseline FDG-PET was not performed on all patients and the treating physician was not blinded to the interim PET/CT results. However,

Table 1
Studies reporting on end-of-treatment FDG-PET results for prediction of progression-free survival

Author, Year Reference	Patient Number	Stage	IPI/aaIPI*	Multicenter	Central Review	Endpoint	PET Criteria	Treatment	Median Follow-Up	EOT PET-CR	PET-CR PFS/EFS	PET-non-CR PFS/EFS	P
Cashen et al,[15] 2011	42	100% III-IV	68% ≥ 3	N	Y	2y PFS 3y PFS	IHP	RCHOP$_{21}$ × 6	34 mo	83%	90%/78%	40%/0%	<.0001
Micallef et al,[16] 2011	81	80% III-IV	77% ≥ 2	Y	Y	3y PFS	Bckg	ER-CHOP	43 m	87%	78%	50%	.02
Cox et al,[17] 2012	85	61% III-IV	83% > 2 RIPI	N	Y	CR, PFS	D 5PS	RCHOP$_{14-21}$ ×6-8 RMACOP	36 mo	87%	90%	58%	.006
Gonzales-Barca et al,[18] 2013	69	65% III-IV	33% ≥ 3	Y	N	3 y EFS	IHP	RCHOP$_{14}$ ×6	29 mo	83%	85%	25%	<.0001
Martelli et al,[19] 2014	115	100% I-II	39% ≥ 3	Y	Y	5y PFS	IHP and D 5PS	MACOP, VACOP, RCHOP$_{14\&21}$	2.9 y	70%	99%	68%	<.0001
Mamot et al,[20] 2015	125	53% III-IV	51% ≥ 2	Y	Y	2y EFS	D 5PS	RCHOP$_{14}$ ×6	24 mo	68%	72%	24%	<.001
Pregno et al,[26] 2012	88	67% III-IV	40% > 3*	N	Y	2y PFS	IHP	RCHOP$_{14-21}$ ×6-8	26 m	88%	83%	64%	<.001
Kanemasa et al,[29] 2017	185	57% III-IV	50% > 3	N	N	5y PFS	IHP	RCHOP or RCHOP-like	37 mo	62%	81%	NA	NA
Kostakoglu et al,[40] 2017	1213	75% III-IV	44% > 2	Y	Y	PFS	D 5PS	RCHOP and GCHOP ×6	29 m	73%	93%	67%	<.0001

Abbreviations: D 5PS, Deauville 5-point scale; EFS, event-free survival; EOT, end of treatment; ER-CHOP, epratuzumab with RCHOP; IHP, International Harmonization Project; IPI, International Prognostic Index; MACOP, methotrexate, leucovorin, doxorubicin, cyclophosphomide, vincristine, perdnisone; N, no; PET-CR, PET–complete remission; PFS, progression-free survival; RIPI, revised IPI; RCHOP, rituximab plus cyclophosphomide, doxorubicin, vincristine, and prednisone; RMACOP, rituximab, methotrexate, leucovorin, doxorubicin, cyclophosphomide, vincristine, perdnisone; Y, yes.

there was no treatment change based on interim PET scans.

In a prospective phase 2 trial testing the safety and efficacy of combining CD22 antibody, epratuzumab with RCHOP (ER-CHOP) in untreated DLBCL, Micallef and colleagues[16] assessed the efficacy of interim PET to predict outcome in DLBCL as a secondary objective. A total of 107 patients were enrolled in the study. All PET scans were centrally reviewed. Overall, 87% of patients (67 of 77) achieved EOT PET-negative status. EOT PET negativity was associated with a statistically significant improvement in EFS ($P = .02$) and OS ($P = .002$). At 3 years, the EFS was 78% if EOT PET was negative compared with 50% if EOT PET was positive. The OS was 90% for EOT PET-negative compared with 50% for EOT PET-positive groups. Similar results were obtained for interim PET after 2 cycles; PET-2 negativity was not associated with a statistically significant improvement in EFS ($P = .31$) or OS ($P = .24$).[16]

Cox and colleagues[17] prospectively evaluated the effectiveness of midtreatment and EOT PET in predicting relapse in a cohort of 85 patients with DLBCL undergoing standard immunochemotherapy. EOT PET was predictive of both PFS and OS, whereas midtreatment PET was predictive of only OS ($P = .013$). In Cox regression, only EOT PET was predictive for both OS ($P = .004$) and PFS ($P = .005$).

In 69 patients with DLBCL who were treated with dose-dense RCHOP, González-Barca and colleagues[18] showed that EOT PET/CT that was interpreted based on IHP criteria predicted EFS. EOT PET/CT was positive in 17.4%, whereas interim PET was positive in 49% of patients. The 3-year EFS was 85.2% for patients with a negative EOT PET and 25% for those with a positive EOT PET ($P<.0001$). In a multivariate analysis including baseline characteristics, interim PET/CT, and EOT PET/CT, EOT PET/CT was the only significant predictor ($P<.0005$). Similar to other reports, the investigators did not find encouraging results of interim PET/CT, which yielded 3-year EFS of 86% for patients who were PET/CT negative versus 64% for those who were PET/CT positive ($P = .036$). The main limitation of this study was that the PET was not centrally reviewed and the interpretation criteria used were IHP criteria which have a known moderate reproducibility shown by several studies using independent evaluations of the same PET scans.[31,32]

Mamot and colleagues[20] prospectively investigated the prognostic value of PET/CT in 138 patients with DLBCL with mixed stages treated with 6 cycles of RCHOP-14 followed by 2 cycles of rituximab. By using central review and the D 5PS, 2-year EFS for EOT PET/CT was 24% (95% CI 9.8%–41.7%) versus 71.5% (95% CI 61.2%–79.5%; $P<.001$) for the PET-positive and PET-negative groups, respectively. Although they demonstrated that the likelihood of 2-year EFS for the interim PET-positive patients was significantly lower than for the PET-negative patients (48% vs. 74%; $P = .004$), the interim PET results were inferior to those of EOT PET results. The predictive value of the quantitative analysis using the ΔSUV_{66} between baseline PET and PET-2 were also inferior ($P = .1$) compared with EOT PET results.

Primary mediastinal large B-cell lymphoma (PMLBCL) is recognized as a distinct entity with clinicopathologic and molecular criteria.[33,34] The response to combination chemotherapy is generally good and is usually followed by consolidation radiotherapy. Similar to DLBCL, if the initial treatment fails, however, the results of salvage chemotherapy and myeloablative treatment are poor. The need to maximize cure rates with initial therapy has led to controversy over its extent; in particular, whether consolidation radiation therapy to the mediastinum is always required and whether PET/CT can be used to determine this. In a study of 115 patients, using D 5P scale and central review, Martelli and colleagues[19] reported that EOT PET-CR after chemoimmunotherapy predicted higher 5-year PFS (98% vs 82%; $P = .0044$) and OS (100% v 91%; $P = .0298$). At EOT, 47% achieved a complete metabolic response (CMR). Using the liver uptake as cutoff for PET positivity discriminated most effectively between high or low risk of failure, with 5-year PFS of 99% versus 68% ($P<.001$) and 5-year OS of 100% versus 83% ($P<.001$). More than 90% of patients are projected to be alive and progression-free at 5 years, despite a low CMR rate (47%) after chemoimmunotherapy. This study provides a basis for using PET/CT to define the role of radiation therapy in PMLBCL.[19]

In summary, these prospective studies collectively confirmed the strong predictive value of EOT FDG-PET for PFS and OS in patients with DLBCL undergoing induction chemotherapy. It is now a routine practice to perform EOT PET scans in all patients with DLBCL either in a clinical trial or routine management setting. Further prospective evidence may be necessary from large phase 3 studies to support the use of PET-CR as an acceptable endpoint for registrational studies.

Retrospective Studies Supporting a Role for Surrogacy for PET–Complete Response

In a pioneering study, Juweid and colleagues[21] retrospectively reported a more accurate assessment of response in a small cohort of 54 patients with aggressive NHL and treated with CHOP in the pre-rituximab era. The investigators evaluated EOT PET by both the International Workshop Criteria (IWC) alone and with incorporating PET into the IWC response criteria (IWC-PET). The definition of PET positivity was based on the mediastinal blood pool (MBP) as the reference site. These PET interpretation criteria, so-called IHP yielded a statistically significant improvement in 3-year PFS compared with those who failed to achieve EOT PET-CR (80% vs 58%, respectively. This study, although with a small sample size, led to the revision of response criteria with incorporation of IHP criteria.[4]

In another cohort of 88 patients with DLBCL who received RCHOP therapy, Pregno and colleagues[26] retrospectively showed a significant correlation between EOT PET results and PFS (EOT PET-CR vs non-CR HR 0.17; 95% CI 0.06–0.46). All PET studies were interpreted with a central review panel according to IHP criteria. In the same study, interim PET scan results correlated poorly with PFS EOT PET/CT (P = .0475). With a median follow-up of 26.2 months, 2-year PFS were 83% in the PET-CR versus 64% in the non–PET-CR groups (P<.001). EOT PET (HR 4.54) and International Prognostic Index (HR = 5.36, P = .001) remained independent prognostic factors.

Traditionally, the International Prognostic Index (IPI) has been used to predict prognosis in patients with DLBCL,[35] and this risk model retained its predictive value in the rituximab era.[36] Both IPI score and the later modifications to the IPI (eg, revised IPI, R-IPI), did not succeed to accurately discriminate the patients at highest risk of relapse beyond 50% for 5-year OS.[37] The more recently proposed scoring system, the National Comprehensive Cancer Network IPI (NCCN-IPI) appeared to improve risk stratification in de novo DLBCL by allowing significantly superior discrimination of both low-risk and high-risk groups, as compared with the traditional IPI.[38] Although PET-CR is widely used as response tool for DLBCL, its prognostic value remains to be better defined. To address this paucity in the literature, Bishton and colleagues[28] retrospectively investigated the value of the NCCN-IPI in a population-based cohort of 223 patients with DLBCL treated with RCHOP or RCHOP-like therapy, and analyzed clinical outcomes with centrally reviewed EOT PET-CT. Consistent with the published NCCN-IPI training and validation series,[38] this study confirmed the superiority of NCCN-IPI over the R-IPI for identifying patients at a very high risk of disease relapse. When the effects of treatment response were

considered, EOT PET-CR was highly predictive of outcome; 5-year OS of 75% versus 36% for those who achieved a PET-CR versus those who did not. Notably, the patients in the worst risk group according to NCCN-IPI experienced the worst outcome regardless of achievement of an EOT PET-CR or CT-CR following RCHOP/ RCHOP-like therapy. By contrast, NCCN-IPI low-risk and intermediate-risk patients achieving a PET-CR experienced 5-year PFS and OS between 76% and 94%. By contrast, the same risk group of patients achieving a CT-CR had 5-year OS and PFS between 76.0% and 81.5%. EOT PET-CR when combined with NCCN-IPI risk groups, conferred a superior power in predicting clinical outcome. In summary, these data suggest that the combination of the NCCN-IPI and PET-CR to RCHOP/CHOP-like therapies is highly predictive of outcome in de novo DLBCL and should be considered as an integrated prognostic system for clinical trials and routine management of patients with DLBCL.

More recently, Kanemasa and colleagues[29] reported similar findings in a series of 185 patients with DLBCL who were treated with RCHOP or an RCHOP-like regimen. Not surprisingly, 114 patients achieved a PET-CR compared with only 71 patients who had a CT-CR. Patients with EOT PET-CR had significantly longer OS and PFS than those with CR by CT only (5-year OS, 87.5 vs 62.4%, P = .003; 5-year PFS, 81.4 vs 60.2%, P = .009). This analysis showed that age, stage, LDH, and PET-CR (HR 0.42; 95% CI 0.20–0.89; P = .024) were significantly associated with OS. Patients with a high risk of relapse according to the NCCN-IPI had an unfavorable outcome regardless of achieving a PET-CR (5-year OS, 62%). In contrast, low-risk, low-intermediate-risk, and high-intermediate-risk patients had excellent outcomes (5-year OS, 100%, 89.7%, and 93.5%, respectively). Among patients with a PET- CR, patients with germinal center B-cell (GCB) subtype of DLBCL had significantly better survival than those with non-GCB DLBCL (5-year OS, 96.9 vs 75.5%, P = .039). These results demonstrated that EOT PET-CR was a better predictor of survival than CR by CT only. The NCCN-IPI and COO subtypes also significant factors to identify a subpopulation of poor-risk patients among those who achieved CR by PET-CT.[29]

Phase III clinical trials provide the most internally valid evidence for studying effects of any testing or intervention to establish or validate an end result. In a retrospective evaluation of a large, prospective, multicenter phase III trial,[39] Kostakoglu and colleagues[40] proved EOT PET-CR to be an effective predictor of PFS in previously untreated patients with DLBCL using both IHP and Lugano criteria. After a median follow-up of 29 months, EOT PET-CR was highly predictive of PFS and highly predictive of OS. The 2.5-year PFS from EOT was significantly higher in patients with PET-CR versus those with non–PET-CR (HR 0.26; 95% CI 0.19–0.38; $P<.0001$). These results were consistent with previously reported studies indicating that EOT PET-CR could be used as an independent prognostic factor for relapse or progression in patients with DLBCL undergoing first-line therapy.[20,28,29]

Molecular gene expression profiling of DLBCL identified at least 3 molecularly distinct forms of DLBCL: the GCB, activated B-cell (ABC or non-GCB), and primary mediastinal B-cell subtypes.[41] Patients with ABC DLBCL have a significantly worse outcome when treated with standard RCHOP chemotherapy.[42] In the published clinical study of GOYA, the results suggested that the GCB subtype was associated with a better outcome than the ABC or unclassified subtypes irrespective of the treatment arm.[39] In the EOT PET/CT imaging analysis, there was suggestion that PFS was higher in patients with a PET-CR versus non–PET-CR independent of COO (unpublished data). Therefore, EOT PET-CR can be used as a surrogate of ultimate outcome in both GCB and ABC subtypes of patients with DLBCL.[40]

THE DEAUVILLE 5-POINT SCALE FOR END-OF-TREATMENT PET ASSESSMENT

The lymphoma response assessment guidelines incorporate both metabolic and anatomic measurements of residual masses to report a response category.[2] Although anatomic disease measurements are also important for determination of PR, SD, and progressive disease, FDG-PET findings usually determine the response categories. The presence of no abnormal FDG uptake is classified as PET-CR, regardless of a residual mass. The 2007 IWG response criteria use the IHP interpretation guidelines for PET-based response assessment.[4] According to these criteria, FDG uptake should be less than the MBP for lesions larger than 2 cm or the adjacent background for smaller lesions to define a PET-CR at the end of treatment.[4,30] In fact, the treatment response is a continuous process and should be registered on a continuous scale rather than in a dichotomous scheme. The response criteria have evolved over the years from a dichotomous reading approach using the adjacent background to D 5PS, which introduced a categorical reading criteria that is better suited to different depth of response.[43,44] The D 5PS scale makes use of the internal reference tissues within the individual patient with a scale ranging from 1 to 5. The liver is the main reference organ that determines the positive (scores 4 or 5) or negative result (scores 1–3) and the MBP determines the categories of negative results (**Box 1**), that is, EOT PET-CR. EOT CMR is represented by scores 1 to 3 regardless of a persistent mass on CT.

The D 5PS has been shown to provide a more reproducible measure of metabolic response with a good interobserver agreement (Cohen's kappa coefficient $[\kappa] = 0.66-0.91$) on assessment of PET-CR.[44–47] These results were comparable with or better than other tumor radiographic response assessment tools, such as Response Evaluation Criteria in Solid Tumors ($\kappa = 0.53-0.63$).[48,49] Because of the favorable aspects of D 5PS, the current guidelines have now incorporated these criteria to assess response as the preferred criteria in patients with lymphoma (Lugano Classification and RECIL).[5,50]

Several investigators have demonstrated the superiority of D 5PS to IHP criteria in EOT PET interpretation using a cutoff of greater than 3 for a positive result (ie, uptake above the normal liver) as compared with score >2 as a cutoff used for the IHP criteria.[19,20,25,51]

Manohar and colleagues[25] retrospectively compared the accuracy of IHP and D 5PS for predicting outcome in 69 patients with aggressive NHL who underwent an EOT FDG-PET/CT and were followed for a minimum period of 12 months (median 17 months).[25] D 5PS criteria better distinguished outcome between patients with positive versus negative scans than the IHP criteria. The 2-year EFS was 85% for PET-CR and 20% for non–PET-CR group ($P<.0001$) compared with 82% and 40% in the respective groups using IHP criteria ($P = .001$). The major difference in accuracy was due to the low positive predictive value of IHP criteria (79.3%vs 88.5%) ($P<.001$). NPVs were similar.

Box 1
Deauville 5-point scale for PET interpretation

1. No uptake

2. Uptake ≤ mediastinum

3. Uptake > mediastinum but ≤ liver

4. Uptake moderately higher than liver

5. Uptake markedly higher than liver and/or new lesions

X. New areas of uptake unlikely to be related to lymphoma

More recently, in a prospective study, Mamot and colleagues[20] demonstrated that the prognostic value of D 5PS was superior to that of IHP in 138 patients with DLBCL who underwent RCHOP treatment. EOT PET interpreted with D 5PS criteria better correlated with EFS than with IHP criteria. The 2-year EFS were 24.0% (95% CI 9.8%–41.7%) versus 39% (95% CI 9.8%–41.7%), respectively, for EOT PET–positive group and 71.5% (95% CI 61.2%–79.5%) and 68% (95% CI 57.1%–76.6%), respectively, for EOT PET-negative group.

In a prospective trial conducted by Martelli and colleagues,[19] 115 patients with PMLBCL EOT PET/CT studies were centrally reviewed after completion of standard chemoimmunotherapy. CMR defined by IHP criteria (score ≤ 2) predicted a 5-year PFS of 98% versus 82% ($P = .004$) and OS of 100% versus 91% ($P = .0298$). However, using liver uptake as cutoff (score >3), as defined by D 5PS, for PET positivity discriminated most effectively between high or low risk of failure, with 5-year PFS of 99% versus 68% ($P<.001$) and 5-year OS of 100% versus 83% ($P<.001$).

SUMMARY

EOT PET-CR is a strong predictor of PFS and OS in DLBCL after first-line immunochemotherapy, using Lugano response criteria or IHP criteria independent of IPI score and COO. Hence, EOT PET-CR is a promising prognostic marker in DLBCL, which has a potential to supersede PFS as a surrogate endpoint in clinical trials. The development of PET-CR as an endpoint may allow for early efficacy interim analysis to expedite and shorten the duration of phase3 trials and clinical development. Nonetheless, further analysis evidence from frontline trials as well meta-analysis of large, prospective, controlled data sets is necessary to better understand the quantitative relation between PET-CR rates and PFS allowing for adequate application of surrogacy.

REFERENCES

1. Gisselbrecht C, Glass B, Mounier N, et al. Salvage regimens with autologous transplantation for relapsed large B-cell lymphoma in the rituximab era. J Clin Oncol 2010;28:4184–90 [Erratum appears in J Clin Oncol 2012;30:1896].
2. Available at: https://www.fda.gov/downloads/Drugs/Guidances/ucm071590.pdf. Accessed February 3, 2019.
3. Maurer MJ, Habermann TM, Shi Q, et al. Progression-free survival at 24 months (PFS24) and subsequent outcome for patients with diffuse large B-cell lymphoma (DLBCL) enrolled on randomized clinical trials. Ann Oncol 2018;29(8):1822–7.
4. Cheson BD, Pfistner B, Juweid ME, et al. Revised response criteria for malignant lymphoma. J Clin Oncol 2007;25:579–86.
5. Cheson BD, Fisher RI, Barrington SF, et al. Recommendations for initial evaluation, staging, and response assessment of Hodgkin and non-Hodgkin lymphoma: the Lugano classification. J Clin Oncol 2014;32:3059–68.
6. Barrington SF, Mikhaeel NG, Kostakoglu L, et al. Role of imaging in the staging and response assessment of lymphoma: consensus of the international conference on malignant lymphomas imaging working group. J Clin Oncol 2014;32:3048–58.
7. Jerusalem G, Beguin Y, Fassotte MF, et al. Whole-body positron emission tomography using 18F-fluorodeoxyglucose for posttreatment evaluation in Hodgkin's disease and non-Hodgkin's lymphoma has higher diagnostic and prognostic value than classical computed tomography scan imaging. Blood 1999;94:429–33.
8. Mikhaeel NG, Timothy AR, O'Doherty MJ, et al. 18-FDG-PET as a prognostic indicator in the treatment of aggressive Non-Hodgkin's Lymphoma-comparison with CT. Leuk Lymphoma 2000;39:543–53.
9. Raanani P, Shasha Y, Perry C, et al. Is CT scan still necessary for staging in Hodgkin and non-Hodgkin lymphoma patients in the PET/CT era? Ann Oncol 2006;17:117–22.
10. Sasaki M, Kuwabara Y, Koga H, et al. Clinical impact of whole body FDG-PET on the staging and therapeutic decision making for malignant lymphoma. Ann Nucl Med 2002;16:337–45.
11. Buchmann I, Reinhardt M, Elsner K, et al. 2-(Fluorine-18)fluoro-2-deoxy-D glucose positron emission tomography in the detection and staging of malignant lymphoma. A bicenter trial. Cancer 2001;91:889–99.
12. Elstrom R, Leonard JP, Coleman M, et al. Combined PET and low-dose, noncontrast CT scanning obviates the need for additional diagnostic contrast-enhanced CT scans in patients undergoing staging or restaging for lymphoma. Ann Oncol 2008;19:1770–3.
13. Luminari S, Biasoli I, Arcaini L, et al. The use of FDG-PET in the initial staging of 142 patients with follicular lymphoma: a retrospective study from the FOLL05 randomized trial of the Fondazione Italiana Linfomi. Ann Oncol 2013;24:2108–12.
14. Zhu Y, Lu J, Wei X, et al. The predictive value of interim and final [18F] fluorodeoxyglucose positron emission tomography after rituximab-chemotherapy in the treatment of non-Hodgkin's lymphoma: a meta-analysis. Biomed Res Int 2013;2013:275805.
15. Cashen AF, Dehdashti F, Luo J, et al. 18F-FDG PET/CT for early response assessment in diffuse large

B-cell lymphoma: poor predictive value of international harmonization project interpretation. J Nucl Med 2011;52(3):386–92.

16. Micallef IN, Maurer MJ, Wiseman GA, et al. Epratuzumab with rituximab, cyclophosphamide, doxorubicin, vincristine, and prednisone chemotherapy in patients with previously untreated diffuse large B-cell lymphoma. Blood 2011;118(15):4053–61.

17. Cox MC, Ambrogi V, Lanni V, et al. Use of interim [18F]fluorodeoxyglucose-positron emission tomography is not justified in diffuse large B-cell lymphoma during first-line immunochemotherapy. Leuk Lymphoma 2012;53(2):263–9.

18. González-Barca E, Canales M, Cortés M, et al. Predictive value of interim 18F-FDG-PET/CT for event-free survival in patients with diffuse large B-cell lymphoma homogenously treated in a phase II trial with six cycles of R-CHOP-14 plus pegfilgrastim as first-line treatment. Nucl Med Commun 2013;34(10):946–52.

19. Martelli M, Ceriani L, Zucca E, et al. [18F]fluorodeoxyglucose positron emission tomography predicts survival after chemoimmunotherapy for primary mediastinal large B-cell lymphoma: results of the International Extranodal Lymphoma Study Group IELSG-26 Study. J Clin Oncol 2014;32(17):1769–75.

20. Mamot C, Klingbiel D, Hitz F, et al. Final results of a prospective evaluation of the predictive value of interim positron emission tomography in patients with diffuse large B-Cell lymphoma treated with R-CHOP-14 (SAKK38/07). J Clin Oncol 2015;33:2523–9.

21. Juweid ME, Wiseman GA, Vose JM, et al. Response assessment of aggressive non-Hodgkin's lymphoma by integrated International Workshop Criteria and fluorine-18-fluorodeoxyglucose positron emission tomography. J Clin Oncol 2005;23:4652–61.

22. Han HS, Escalon MP, Hsiao B, et al. High incidence of false-positive PET scans in patients with aggressive non-Hodgkin's lymphoma treated with rituximab-containing regimens. Ann Oncol 2009;20:309–18.

23. Phan J, Mazloom A, Medeiros LJ, et al. Benefit of consolidative radiation therapy in patients with diffuse large B-cell lymphoma treated with R-CHOP chemotherapy. J Clin Oncol 2010;28:4170–6.

24. Yoo C, Lee DH, Kim JE, et al. Limited role of interim PET/CT in patients with diffuse large B-cell lymphoma treated with R-CHOP. Ann Hematol 2011;90(7):797–802.

25. Manohar K, Mittal BR, Raja S, et al. Comparison of various criteria in interpreting end of therapy F-18 labeled fluorodeoxyglucose positron emission tomography/computed tomography in patients with aggressive non-Hodgkin lymphoma. Leuk Lymphoma 2013;54(4):714–9.

26. Pregno P, Chiappella A, Bello M, et al. Interim 18-FDG-PET/CT failed to predict the outcome in diffuse large B-cell lymphoma patients treated at the diagnosis with rituximab-CHOP. Blood 2012;119:2066–73.

27. Adams HJ, de Klerk JM, Fijnheer R, et al. Residual anatomical disease in diffuse large B-cell lymphoma patients with FDG-PET-based complete response after first-line R-CHOP therapy: does it have any prognostic value? J Comput Assist Tomogr 2015;39:810–5.

28. Bishton MJ, Hughes S, Richardson F, et al. Delineating outcomes of patients with diffuse large B cell lymphoma using the National Comprehensive Cancer Network-International Prognostic Index and positron emission tomography-defined remission status; a population-based analysis. Br J Haematol 2016;172:246–54.

29. Kanemasa Y, Shimoyama T, Sasaki Y, et al. Analysis of prognostic value of complete response by PET-CT and further stratification by clinical and biological markers in DLBCL patients. Med Oncol 2017;34(2):29.

30. Juweid ME, Stroobants S, Hoekstra OS, et al. Use of positron emission tomography for response assessment of lymphoma: consensus of the Imaging Subcommittee of International Harmonization Project in Lymphoma. J Clin Oncol 2007;25:571–8.

31. Horning SJ, Juweid ME, Schoder H, et al. Interim positron emission tomography scans in diffuse large B-cell lymphoma: an independent expert nuclear medicine evaluation of the Eastern Cooperative Oncology Group E3404 study. Blood 2010;115:775–7 [quiz: 918].

32. Thomas A, Gingrich RD, Smith BJ, et al. 18-Fluorodeoxyglucose positron emission tomography report interpretation as predictor of outcome in diffuse large B-cell lymphoma including analysis of 'indeterminate' reports. Leuk Lymphoma 2010;51:439–46.

33. Steidl C, Gascoyne RD. The molecular pathogenesis of primary mediastinal large B-cell lymphoma. Blood 2011;118:2659–69.

34. Johnson PW, Davies AJ. Primary mediastinal B-cell lymphoma. Hematol Am Soc Hematol Educ Program 2008;349-358.

35. The International Non-Hodgkin's Lymphoma Prognostic Factors Project. A predictive model for aggressive non-Hodgkin's lymphoma. The international non-Hodgkin's lymphoma prognostic factors project. N Engl J Med 1993;329:987–94.

36. Ziepert M, Hasenclever D, Kuhnt E, et al. Standard International Prognostic Index remains a valid predictor of outcome for patients with aggressive CD20+ B-cell lymphoma in the rituximab era. J Clin Oncol 2010;28:2373–80.

37. Sehn LH, Berry B, Chhanabhai M, et al. The revised International Prognostic Index (R-IPI) is a better

predictor of outcome than the standard IPI for patients with diffuse large B-cell lymphoma treated with R-CHOP. Blood 2007;109:1857–61.

38. Zhou Z, Sehn LH, Rademaker AW, et al. An enhanced International Prognostic Index (NCCN-IPI) for patients with diffuse large B-cell lymphoma treated in the rituximab era. Blood 2014;123:837–42.

39. Vitolo U, Trněný M, Belada D, et al. Obinutuzumab or rituximab plus cyclophosphamide, doxorubicin, vincristine, and prednisone in previously untreated diffuse large B-cell lymphoma. J Clin Oncol 2017; 35:3529–37.

40. Kostakoglu, Martelli M, Sehn LH, et al. End of treatment PET-CT predicts progression free survival in DLBCL after first-line treatment: results from the Phase III GOYA study. 14th International Conference on Malignant Lymphoma (14-ICML). Lugano, Switzerland (abstr), June 14–17, 2017.

41. Alizadeh AA, Eisen MB, Davis RE, et al. Distinct types of diffuse large B-cell lymphoma identified by gene expression profiling. Nature 2000;403: 503–11.

42. Rosenwald A, Wright G, Chan WC, et al. The use of molecular profiling to predict survival after chemotherapy for diffuse large-B-cell lymphoma. N Engl J Med 2002;346:1937–47.

43. Meignan M, Gallamini A, Haioun C. Report on the first international Workshop on interim-PET scan in lymphoma. Leuk Lymphoma 2009;50:1257–60.

44. Barrington SF, Qian W, Somer EJ, et al. Concordance between four European centres of PET reporting criteria designed for use in multicentre trials in Hodgkin lymphoma. Eur J Nucl Med Mol Imaging 2010;37:1824–33.

45. Le Roux PY, Gastinne T, Le Gouill S, et al. Prognostic value of interim FDG PET/CT in Hodgkin's lymphoma patients treated with interim response-adapted strategy: comparison of International Harmonization Project (IHP), Gallamini and London criteria. Eur J Nucl Med Mol Imaging 2011;38(6):1064–71.

46. Furth C, Amthauer H, Hautzel H, et al. Evaluation of interim PET response criteria in paediatric Hodgkin's lymphoma-results for dedicated assessment criteria in a blinded dual-centre read. Ann Oncol 2011;22: 1198–203.

47. Itti E, Meignan M, Berriolo-Riedinger A, et al. An international confirmatory study of the prognostic value of early PET/CT in diffuse large B-cell lymphoma: comparison between Deauville criteria and ΔSUVmax. Eur J Nucl Med Mol Imaging 2013;40: 1312–20.

48. Suzuki C, Torkzad MR, Jacobsson H, et al. Interobserver and intraobserver variability in the response evaluation of cancer therapy according to RECIST and WHO-criteria. Acta Oncol 2010;49(4):509–14.

49. Sato Y, Watanabe H, Sone M, et al. Tumor response evaluation criteria for HCC (hepatocellular carcinoma) treated using TACE (transcatheter arterial chemoembolization): RECIST (response evaluation criteria in solid tumors) version 1.1 and mRECIST (modified RECIST): JIVROSG-0602. Ups J Med Sci 2013;118:16–22.

50. Younes A, Hilden P, Coiffier B, et al. International Working Group consensus response evaluation criteria in lymphoma (RECIL 2017). Ann Oncol 2017;28:1436–47.

51. Dupuis J, Berriolo-Riedinger A, Julian A, et al. Impact of [18F]fluorodeoxyglucose positron emission tomography response evaluation in patients with high-tumor burden follicular lymphoma treated with immunochemotherapy: a prospective study from the Groupe d'Etudes des Lymphomes de l'Adulte and GOELAMS. J Clin Oncol 2012;30: 4317–22.

PET-Derived Quantitative Metrics for Response and Prognosis in Lymphoma

Lale Kostakoglu, MD, MPH[a],*, Stéphane Chauvie, PhD[b]

KEYWORDS

• Lymphoma • FDG-PET • Quantitative metrics • Response • Prognosis

KEY POINTS

- Diffuse large B-cell lymphoma (DLBCL) is a highly heterogeneous disease with clinicopathologic and genotypic diversity. Although it is potentially curable, most patients whose disease relapses within the first 2 years of first-line treatment have a significantly inferior survival.
- End of therapy (EOT) PET-CR is an independent predictor of PFS and OS in DLBCL after first-line immunochemotherapy, using Lugano response criteria.
- The development of PET-CR as an endpoint, replacing PFS, may allow for early efficacy interim analysis to expedite and shorten the duration of clinical trials and clinical development of novel therapeutics.
- Meta-analysis of large, prospective, controlled data sets is necessary to better understand the relation between PET-CR rates and PFS allowing for adequate application of surrogacy.

SEMIQUANTITATIVE PARAMETERS IN PET WITH FLUDEOXYGLUCOSE

Among the different metrics that are used to describe tumor burden and tumor metabolic activity, metabolic tumor volume (MTV) and total lesion glycolysis (TLG) have become favorite topics on which the scientific community concentrated in the recent years.[1] Indeed, the standardized uptake value (SUV), defined as the ratio of the decay corrected fludeoxyglucose (FDG) concentration in a volume of interest (VOI) to the injected dose normalized to the patient's body weight, even if very well-known from the beginning of PET era, never emerged as an index clearly holding a predictive or prognostic role in lymphoma. Besides, the maximum SUV value in a region (SUV_{max}), it is often reported in everyday clinical practice in PET referral as an additional descriptor of the FDG avidity of single lesions. One of the major complications in the use of SUV_{max} is that it is significantly influenced by tumor heterogeneity and image noise because is measured in a single voxel. This factor leads to high fluctuation of its values and its position within the high-uptake region of a lesion. Consequently, repeated tumor SUV_{max} measurements may show an intrapatient bias of 5% to 30%.[2] To decrease the dependency of SUV on image noise, an alternative figure of merit, SUV_{peak}, representing the maximum tumor activity within a 1 cm³ VOI in the high-uptake part of the lesion[3–5] has been proposed. SUV_{peak}, being averaged over a larger number of voxels, is less prone to fluctuation and its position remains stable in the hottest part of the tumor. Indeed, SUV_{peak} yields less intrapatient bias (1% to 11%) compared with SUV_{max}.[2] Nevertheless, a recent study that compared SUV_{max} and SUV_{peak} found that different SUV definitions yielded a 20% variation in tumor response values for an individual tumor and variation of up to 90% for a single SUV measurement.[6]

To account for the varying biodistribution of FDG in different body compositions, in addition

[a] Nuclear Medicine and Molecular Imaging, Department of Radiology, Icahn School of Medicine at Mount Sinai, One Gustave L. Levy Place, Box 1141, New York, NY 10029, USA; [b] Department of Medical Physics, 'Santa Croce e Carle' Hospital, Cuneo, Italy
* Corresponding author.
E-mail address: Lale.kostakoglu@mssm.edu

PET Clin 14 (2019) 317–329
https://doi.org/10.1016/j.cpet.2019.03.002
1556-8598/19/© 2019 Elsevier Inc. All rights reserved.

to body weight–based SUV, other SUV indices have also been proposed.[3,7,8] One of this is SUL, that is, SUV normalized to lean body mass, which take in account for the poor FDG uptake in fat. To account for both the aforementioned physical and biological factors, SUL_{peak} has been proposed as measurement for therapy response in PET Response Criteria in Solid Tumors (PERCIST).[5]

MEASUREMENT OF METABOLICALLY ACTIVE TUMOR VOLUME

MTV and TLG are SUV-based derived PET metrics,[9–11] and both measure metabolically active tumor tissue within the entire tumor mass that can encompass the entire body, reflecting tumor functionality. By definition, the MTV determines the total volume in a VOI, and thus, is expressed in cubic centimeters or milliliters. The TLG is the product of the SUV_{mean} within the drawn VOI and the MTV, representing an index that includes the tumor volume and the average uptake of the entire tumor.

These indices heavily rely on the definition of a VOI that univocally identifies the tumor volume. This requires 2 stages: (1) the exact definition of the lesion where the VOI is delineated and (2) the segmentation of each lesion to define the borders of the VOI, even if the first stage would be better performed using an automated method with an advanced software. The majority of available softwares require an imaging expert intervention for manual correction of the erroneously included physiologic sites within the VOIs. There are 2 basic ways of doing this task, by defining each lesion individually (point picking) or by defining a gross region that contains 1 or more lesions. In the second stage, then, the VOIs of the tumors are defined by segmentation, a process that identifies which voxel belongs to the tumor of interest, segregating it from the surrounding tissue.

A multitude of segmentation algorithms have been described in the literature but, as of now, there is no consensus on the optimal or most accurate algorithm, and hence, there is no universally accepted reproducible and practical method for segmentation. The comparison of different segmentation methods is challenging,[11–19] because a ground truth does not exist. The variability in MTV delineation by different segmentation algorithms has been reported in the range of 40% to 400%.[11,12,18,19] Indeed, the performance of tumor delineation methods heavily depends on the shape and dimension signal to background ratio of the tumor itself, rendering it mostly impossible to identify a one-size-fits-all algorithm. Advanced techniques have also been developed to overcome the challenges associated with other thresholding methodologies,[20,21] but their reproducibility

remains questionable. Thresholding, both with a fixed threshold (SUV_{max} of 2.5 or SUV_{max} of 4.0) or with a percentage threshold, that is, 25% or 42% of the SUV_{max}, is the most widely used algorithm in lymphoma studies. This method is mostly implemented by commercially or publicly available softwares; its intrinsic simplicity and its acceptable reproducibility. But it is clear that these 2 distinct methodologies provide dramatically different results for MTVs either on a single lesion, or a single patient basis. Consequently, the average and median MTV calculated in the same patient population are dramatically different, as discussed in Clinical Applications of Quantitative PET in Lymphoma, that renders very difficult the usage of cutoffs obtained with predictive statistical analysis.

It is widely established that the SUV_{max} is significantly affected by host-specific biological and imaging-related physical and technical factors. Mostly, all the authors demonstrating an added value of SUV-derived metrics to image interpretation emphasized that validation of PET-computed tomography (CT) findings under standardized circumstances is essential. In recent years, guidelines for standardization guidelines of PET-CT imaging for oncologic studies have been proposed by a group of physicians and scientists associated with the European Association of Nuclear Medicine, and the Society of Nuclear Medicine.[7] These guidelines were developed to achieve consistency for SUVs across multiple centers and also require cross-calibration of the PET scanners and dose calibrators to tune in the image reconstruction algorithm to achieve an optimal curve for recovery coefficient. This painstaking approach decrease interscanner variability of the measured activity to 5% to 10%.[22–25] Based on the results of the recent studies, protocol variation should be kept to a minimum when performing repeat scans to improve the reproducibility of SUV measurements.

Clinical Applications of Quantitative PET in Lymphoma

Continuous quantitative metrics as provided by PET-derived quantitative analysis provides a relatively more accurate means to determine tumor burden and assess treatment-related metabolic changes in a finer scale compared with traditional dichotomous response categorization. The MTV as a measure of the viable tumor fraction or TLG as a product of MTV and the mean SUV within the metabolically active tumor volume, has the potential to decrease the rate of false-positive results attendant with existing qualitative methods, increase reproducibility, and maximize statistical power in the prediction of survival. With the recent

Table 1
Studies investigating the prognostic value of with MTV in HL, DLBCL, PMBCL

Reference	Patients Population	No. of Patients	Study Design	Multi center	Mono, Multi, or Equalized Scanners	Therapy	PET Timing	Segmentation Method	Segmentation Performed by	Cutoff Values
Song et al,[36]	Early HL	127	RE	Yes	MU	6 × ABVD + 30 Gy of IFRT + 10 Gy on initial bulky	Baseline	Visual and threshold of 2.5 SUV	Locally, reviewed centrally by an expert	MTV = 198 cm^3
Kanoun et al,[37]	HL	59	RE	No	MU (2 scanners)	4-6 cycles of an anthracycline-based chemotherapy + 20-36 Gy of IFRT	Baseline, interim	Threshold 41% SUV_{max} manually adjusted	2 blinded experts, consensus if discrepant	MTV = 225 cm^3
Tseng et al,[33]	Early and advanced HL	30	RE	No	MO	Stanford V, ABVD, VAMP, or BEACOPP + RT (20, 25.5, or 36 Gy)	Baseline, interim	Region-growing algorithm	—	Not significant
Cottereau et al,[38]	Early HL	258	PRO	Yes	MU	89.5% ABVD	Baseline, interim	Threshold 41% SUV_{max} manually adjusted	expert	MTV = 147 mL
Akhtari et al,[39]	Early	267	PRO	NO	MO	ABVD + INRT (30 Gy)	Baseline, interim	Threshold of 2.5 SUV		MTV = 268 mL, TLG = 1703 mL
Moskowitz A et al,[41]	Relapsed and refractory HL	65	PRO	No	MO	BV, AugICE + ASCT	Baseline, interim	Threshold 41% SUV_{max} manually adjusted		MTV = 109.5 mL
Hussien et al,[35]	Pediatric HL	54	PRO	Yes	EQ	GPOH-HD2002P, GPOH-HD2003, EuroNet-PHL-C1 plus IFRT	Baseline, interim	Threshold of 2.5 SUV (body-weight, body surface) and threshold of mean liver plus 2 SD of SUV (lean body mass)	Two blinded experts	MTV = 0 TLG = 0.3 ΔMTV = 99.99% ΔTGV = 99.95% @interim
Rogash et al,[44]	Pediatric HL	50	PRO	Yes	EQ	Two cycles of induction chemotherapy (OEPA) before ERA				
Kim et al,[48]	DLBCL	140	RE	No	MO	6-8 cycles of R-CHOP + 36 Gy of RT bulky disease	Baseline	Visual and threshold at 25%, 50%, and 75% of SUV_{max}	Three experts	TLG = 415.5 at 50% of SUV_{max}

(continued on next page)

Table 1
(continued)

Reference	Patients Population	No. of Patients	Study Design	Multi center	Mono, Multi, or Equalized Scanners	Therapy	PET Timing	Segmentation Method	Segmentation Performed by	Cutoff Values
Sasanelli et al,[47]	DLBCL	114	RE	Yes	MU	R-CHOP21, RCHOP14, and ASCT	Baseline	Threshold 41% of SUV_{max}	One expert, subset of 50 by another	MTV = 550 cm^3
Song et al,[45]	DLBCL	169	RE	No	MU	6–8 cycles of R-CHOP	Baseline	Threshold of 2.5 SUV	Two experts	MTV = 220 cm^3
Gallicchio et al,[57]	DLBCL	52	RE	No	MO	R-CHOP	Baseline	Visual and threshold of 42% SUV_{max}	Three blinded experts (subsets of 18 patients in double)	MTV = 16.1 cm^3 TLG = 589.5
Adams et al,[50]	DLBCL	73	RE	No	MO, EQ	R-CHOP	Baseline	Threshold of 40% of the SUV_{max}	Single-blinded expert	MTV = 272.3 cm^3 TLG = 2955.4
Zhou et al,[54]	DLBCL	91	RE	Yes	MO	R-CHOP	Baseline	Liver SUV_{mean} plus 3 SD	Two experts	MTV = 70 cm^3 TGV = 826.5
Malek et al,[59]	DLBCL	140	RE	No	MO	R-CHOP or R-DA-EPOCH	Interim (2–4 cycles)	D-5PS, a 37% threshold of SUVmax and a gradient technique method.	One expert	ΔSUV_{max} >72% ΔMTV 52%
Xie et al,[56]	DLBCL	60	RE	No	MO	R-CHOP	Baseline	Threshold liver SUV_{mean} plus 2 SD of liver SUV	Not specified	MTV = 850.3 cm^3 TGV = 4758
Park et al,[71]	DLBCL	100	RE	No	MO	3–8 R-CHOP	Baseline, interim	Threshold MBPS	Two experts	Not given (median?)

Study	Disease	N				Treatment	Timepoint	Threshold method	Reader	Metrics
Mikhaeel et al,[53]	DLBCL	147	PRO	No	MO	4–6 R-CHOP (PET adapted strategy)	Baseline, interim	Threshold SUV = 2.5, manually adjusted	One expert	MTV = 396 cm³
Toledano et al,[58]	DLBCL	114	RE	No	MO	R-CHOP	Baseline	Threshold 41% of SUV_{max}	One expert	MTV = 261 mL
Ceriani et al,[63]	PMBCL	103	PRO	Yes	MU	R-CHOP and R-VACOB-P + IFRT	Baseline	threshold 25% of SUV_{max} manually corrected	One expert centrally	MTV = 703 cm³, TLG 5814
Pinnix et al,[64]	PMBCL	65	RE	No	MO	DA-R-EPOCH	Baseline, EOT	threshold of 25% and 42% of SUV_{max}	One expert centrally	MTV = 323.6 mL TLG = 3941

Abbreviations: ABVD, adriamycin, bleomycin, vinblastine, and dacarbazine; ASCT, autologous stem cell transplantation; augICE, augmented ifosfamide, carboplatin, and etoposide; BEA-COPP, bleomycin, etoposide, adriamycin (doxorubicin), cyclophosphamide, oncovin, procarbazine, prednisone; BV, brentuximab vedotin; DLBCL, diffuse large b-cell lymphoma, IFRT, involved-field radiation therapy; INRT, involved node radiotherapy; MO, mono; MU, multi; PRO, prospective; R-CHOP, rituximab, cyclophosphamide, doxorubicin, vincristine, and prednisolone; R-DA-EPOR, ; RE, retrospective; RT, radiation therapy; R-VACOB-P, ; SD, standard deviation; VAMP, vincristine, doxorubicin hydrochloride (adriamycin), methotrexate and prednisone.

insurgence of advanced software programs, tumor volumes can be now determined without extensive effort, including the recommendations on standardization expressed in Measurement of Metabolically Active Tumor Volume.

PROGNOSTIC VALUE OF TUMOR METABOLIC VOLUME

In an effort to reduce false-positive results using qualitative interpretation methods and better address tumor heterogeneity for proper treatment decisions, the predictive value of PET-based evaluation and volumetric measurements, that is, MTV and TLG have been under investigation in the past several years. There is, however, a paucity of published data on large prospective series to justify a role for pretherapy quantitative PET metrics affecting clinical outcomes of lymphoma patients. The available literature in both Hodgkin lymphoma (HL) and non-Hodgkin lymphoma (NHL) is discussed in the following section and summarized in **Table 1**.

Hodgkin Lymphoma

HL is a potentially curable malignancy with combined modality therapies. Nonetheless, approximately 20% of patients with HL fail to attain a complete remission or they relapse during follow-up.[26] Patients with a bulky disease may need intensive therapy involving high-dose chemotherapy or other alternative treatments. However, the definition of tumor bulk is not standardized or validated and also is traditionally measured using 1 dimension.[27,28] Historically, the extent of disease has been indirectly derived from the number of tumor sites, disease stage, and lactate dehydrogenase levels, all of which are suggestive markers of tumor burden.[29–32] A direct measurement of disease bulk using PET-derived metabolic volumes would be useful as a prognostic surrogate. If validated, the integration of this metric into predictive models may change the strength of contribution of existing parameters in the current risk stratification systems.

Multiple retrospective studies published contrasting results for the role of MTV in mixed populations consisting of patients with early and advanced stage HL.[33–41] In a retrospective analysis of prospectively acquired data in 89 patients with classical HL treated with standard therapy, the typical MTV (TMTV) was found to be the strongest predictor of progression-free survival (PFS) at baseline ($P = .002$) and qualitative analysis using Deauville 5-point scoring(D-5PS) at PET1, at early interim analysis ($P < .0001$).[34] In contrast, Tseng and colleagues[33] reported that baseline PET metrics including SUV_{max} and TMTV did not

predict survival in 30 patients with HL (mostly stages IIB–IV) treated with varying chemotherapy regimens with or without involved-field radiation therapy while the change in MTV (ΔMTV; $P < .01$), change in TLG ($P < .01$), and change is SUV_{max} (ΔSUV_{max}; $P = .02$) at interim PET were associated with PFS and overall survival (OS). These results suggest that the chemosensitivity of the tumor as measured by an early PET study during ongoing treatment may be a better predictor of clinical outcome than the initial tumor bulk. In pediatric patients with HL (n = 54), similar data were published by Hussien and colleagues,[35] who showed that all quantitative PET measures (SUV_{max}, MTV, and TLG) fared significantly better than DS at PET2. However, ΔSUV_{max} was the most powerful predictor of treatment outcome ($P < .001$). These early studies are limited and nongeneralizable, however, because of the small number of cohorts, the inclusion of relapsed patients, and the various chemotherapy regimens used, including intensive treatments.

Song and colleagues[36] showed a high association between TMTV and poor prognosis in a group of 127 patients with early stage HL. With a median follow-up of 52 months and a segmentation cutoff of SUV_{max} of 2.5, the high TMTV (>198 cm^3) status was independently associated with PFS ($P = .008$) and OS ($P = .007$).[36] Several recent publications have also supported these findings, demonstrating a significantly worse prognosis in patients who have a high TMTV at baseline using a segmentation cutoff of 41% SUV_{max}.[37,38] Kanoun and colleagues,[37] in a cohort of 59 patients with HL with mixed stages (stages II–IV), showed that patients with a baseline TMTV of greater than 225 cm^3 had a significantly worse 4-year PFS than those with a low TMTV (42% vs 85%; $P = .001$). Moreover, TMTV had more potent predictive power for outcome than the IPS and the traditional bulk definition (mass of >10 cm). In multivariate analysis only baseline MTV ($P < .006$; relative risk, 4.4) and ΔSUV_{max} at PET2 (71%; $P = .0005$; relative risk, 6.3) remained independent predictors of , although while tumor bulk (>10 cm) did not reach a statistical significance. The combination of the prognostic stratification by TMTV with interim PET allowed an identification of a new patient subset with a distinctly different PFS profile ($P < .0001$).[37]

The retrospective analysis of the standard arm of the H10 Intergroup trial of early stage patients with HL (n = 258; 61% early stage unfavorable [ESU]), by Cottereau and colleagues[38] revealed a 5-year PFS and OS of 71% and 83% in the high TMTV (>147 cm^3) group compared with 92% and 98%, respectively, in the low TMTV group. In a multivariate analysis, TMTV was the only baseline prognosticator compared with the current staging systems.

TMTV and iPET2 were independently prognostic and, the two combined, identified 4 different risk groups with the lowest risk group having a 5-year PFS of 95%, versus 25% for the highest risk group.

In another large cohort of patients with early stage HL (n = 267; 67% ESU), Akhtari and colleagues[39] reported similar findings with a high correlation between MTVs and freedom from progression (FFP). The FFP, dichotomizing with an 80th percentile TMTV cutoff of 268 cm^3 and TLG cutoff of 1703 cm^3, was significantly worse for those with high a TMTV (P = .008) or high TLG (P = .001) than for those with a low MTV or a TLG. These results also corroborated the previously published data by Kanoun and colleagues,[40] who showed that all segmentation methods for TMTV correlated with outcome in patients with HL of all stages. TMTV further subcategorized the ESU HL into 2 groups in which FFP was significantly worse for patients with ESU disease accompanied with a high TMTV (>268 cm^3) or TLG (1703 cm^3) than those with a low TMTV or TLG.[39] On multivariable analysis, after adjusting for traditional risk classification, TMTV (for every 100-unit increase: hazard ratio [HR], 1.14; 95% confidence interval [CI], 1.02–1.26; P = .016) and TLG (for every 500-unit increase: HR, 1.096; 95% CI, 1.00–1.20; P = .047) were strongly associated with FFP. These findings may be significant for clinical trial designs in patients with ESU to further streamline treatment approach with treatment escalation for the high-risk ESU group.

The identification of prognostic factors for patients with relapsed/refractory HL is also as important as newly diagnosed patients, for a risk adapted therapy optimization. In a phase II study of PET-adapted therapy (n = 75) with brentuximab vedotin before autologous stem cell transplantation (ASCT); PET-negative patients (D-5PS ≤ 2) proceeded to ASCT, whereas PET-positive patients received augmented ifosfamide, carboplatin, and etoposide before ASCT.[41] The baseline TMTV (P < .001) and refractory disease (P = .003) were independent prognostic factors for event-free survival (EFS). Low TMTV (<109.5 cm^3; segmentation threshold 41% of the SUV$_{max}$) and relapsed disease identified a favorable group (3-year EFS, 100%). The 3-year EFS rates for patients with low and high MTV were 92% and 27%, respectively (P < .001). TMTV increased the predictive power of PET before ASCT; the 3-year EFS was 86% for pre-ASCT PET-positive patients with a low TMTV.

Despite these encouraging results, it is still premature to start designing clinical trials without standardization of the quantification methods. Further investigations should include an expanded number of patients and prospective, multicenter, homogeneous, large datasets to definitively determine the complementary or independent role of quantitative FDG-PET metrics at baseline for predicting prognosis and guiding treatment decisions in HL.

Diffuse Large B-Cell Lymphoma

Unlike HL, the disease bulk is not a universally accepted prognostic factor for diffuse large b-cell lymphoma (DLBCL).[42] However, there are published data, although limited, suggesting a role for tumor bulk imparting an unfavorable outcome.[42–44] Recently, in an effort to improve the predictive value of PET, TMTV and TLG measurements were investigated as predictors of survival in patients with DLBCL treated with standard therapy consisting of rituximab, cyclophosphamide, doxorubicin, vincristine, and prednisolone (R-CHOP).[45–53] The majority of these data were retrospective and, irrespective of variable segmentation thresholds, most showed a favorable PFS and OS for patients with a low TMTV compared those with a high TMTV based on the cutoff value.[45–53] Sasanelli and colleagues,[47] using a threshold of 41% of the SUV$_{max}$ and a median follow-up of 39 months, demonstrated a prognostic value for TMTV in 114 patients with DLBCL who received R-CHOP (HR, 4.4; P = .008 for PFS and HR, 3.1, P = .049 for OS).[37] The 3-year PFS were 77% and 60% in the low and in the high TMTV groups, respectively (>509 cc^3; P = .04). TMTV was the only independent predictor of OS (P = .002) and PFS (P = .03) compared with other pretherapy indices, including tumor bulk (>10 cm), lactate dehydrogenase, stage, and age-adjusted International Prognostic Index (IPI). Interestingly, the TLG failed to predict PFS and was less predictive of OS than TMTV. This retrospective study, however, was limited by the variability of therapy protocols as well as the lack of comparative analysis between volumetric results and SUVs with respect to the prediction of PFS.

More recently, several studies corroborated an independent predictive value for metabolic tumor measurements with respect to survival.[53,58] In a retrospective single-center study, Mikhaeel and colleagues[53] found that the pretreatment TMTV, using an SUV threshold of 2.5, was the strongest predictor of PFS in 147 patients with DLBCL who were treated with R-CHOP and had a median follow-up of 3.8 years. The optimal cutoff for MTV was 396 cc^3 and Kaplan–Meier survival analysis showed that a high MTV (>400) was associated with a poor outcome (P < .001). At univariate analysis, IPI and TMTV were significant, whereas the SUV$_{max}$ was not, and at multivariate analysis only baseline MTV maintained its prognostic value. Combining baseline MTV and PET2 data interpreted by D-5PS criteria improved the predictive power of interim PET. This analysis segregated the study population into 3 distinct prognostic groups: good (MTV <400; 5-year PFS of >90%), intermediate (MTV ≥400 + DS 1–3; 5-year PFS of 58.5%), and poor (MTV ≥400 + DS 4–5; 5-year PFS of 29.7%). Using the same patient population, the investigators tested the hypothesis that different segmentation cutoffs will not change the prognostic value of metabolic tumor measurements. Proving this hypothesis, the TMTV remained a strong predictor of PFS with all methods having comparable accuracy but with, notably, largely different cutoffs ranging 166 to 400 mL. The segmentation cutoffs included an SUV of 2.5 or greater, an SUV of 41% or greater of the maximum SUV, and an SUV greater than or equal to the mean liver uptake.[5] Investigating the impact of various segmentation methods, Malek and colleagues[59] also observed no difference in the prognostic value of TMTV in a retrospective study of 140 patients with DLBCL. However, these authors showed that a gradient-based method for segmentation led to a statistically significant greater TMTV at pretreatment, as well as interim PET respect to the threshold-based method. In this study, D-5PS did not correlate with PFS and ΔMTV at PET2 was a better predictor of PFS compared with $ΔSUV_{max}$ (area under the curve [AUC], $AUC_{ΔMTV}$ of 0.713 and $AUC_{ΔSUVmax}$ of 0.873; $P = .0324$). Similarly, Zhou and colleagues[54] reported TLG to be the only independent predictor in a population of 91 patients with newly diagnosed DLBCL treated with R-CHOP and followed for a median of 30 months. The metabolic volumes were segmented using the mean liver SUV plus 3 standard deviations. The 5-year PFS for the high and low TLG values were 83% and 34%, respectively ($P < .001$). For the same subgroups the 5-year OS were 92% and 67%, respectively ($P < .001$). The SUV_{max} and DLBCL cell of origin were not found to have a prognostic value. Even in patients with remission, the patients with higher TLG or MTV had more risk of relapse or disease progression.

In an effort to improve the predictive value, Cottereau and colleagues[55] retrospectively analyzed the combination of MTV with molecular signatures including cell of origin (ABC vs GCB subtypes), and high-risk gene (MYC and BCL2) overexpression. A 41% $SUV_{max\ segmentation}$ threshold resulted in a 300 mL cutoff; patients with high MTV had a 5-year PFS and OS of 43% and 46%, respectively, compared with 76% and 78, respectively, for patients with a low MTV ($P = .0023$ and $P = .0047$, respectively). Cell of origin status, MYC, or BCL2 gene overexpression and overexpression of both genes (double expressor) were significantly associated with worse survival. High MTV identified in molecular low-risk patients yielded a group with a very poor outcome (MYC: PFS = 51%, OS = 55%; BCL2: PFS = 49%, OS = 49%; or double expressor: PFS = 50%, OS = 50%) and low MTV predicted a group with a very good outcome (MYC: PFS = 93%, OS = 93%; BCL2: PFS = 86%, OS = 86%; or double expressor: PFS = 81%, OS = 81%). Likewise, Toledano and colleagues[58] reported in a cohort of 114 consecutive DLBCL lymphoma patients, with an optimal MTV cutoff of 261 mL calculated with 41% threshold, a high MTV had a 5-year PFS and OS of 37% and 39%, respectively, in comparison with 72% and 83%, respectively, in patients with a low MTV ($P = .0002$ for PFS; $P < .0001$ for OS). On multivariate analysis, MTV, cell of origin phenotype, and IPI were independent predictive factors for both PFS and OS ($P < .05$ for both). The combination of the GEP and MTV leaded to the identification of 3 sub-risk populations: for patients with a low MTV overall, those with a high TMTV and GCB phenotype, and patients with a high MTV and ABC phenotype, 5-year PFS rates were 72%, 51%, and 17% ($P < .0001$), and 5-year OS rates were 83%, 55%, and 17% ($P < .0001$), respectively.

There are also some contradicting results for the prognostic value of TMTV and TLG.[50,57] In a study of 52 intermediate risk (by IPI) patients with DLBCL treated with R-CHOP and with a median follow-up of 18 months, Gallicchio and colleagues[57] found the SUV_{max} to be a better predictor of EFS ($P = .0002$; HR, 0.13) than TMTV and TLG. Likewise, Adams and colleagues[50] retrospectively showed the superiority for NCCN-IPI as predictor of survival compared with TMTV and TLG in 73 patients with DLBCL ($P = .024$).[50,60] Although these studies authors used a similar threshold (40%–42% of SUV_{max}) for segmentation, the significantly divergent results from prior published data might be on the account of inadequate sample size and methodologic differences.

A systematic review of 7 retrospective studies in 703 patients with DLBCL[56] suggested that both SUV_{max} and MTV have significant prognostic value for PFS (HR, 1.61 [$P = .038$] and HR, 2.18 [$P = .000$], respectively). The high 3-year OS is unfavorably impacted by high MTV and TLG values (odds ratios of 5.40 and 2.19, respectively). However, the use of different risk scoring systems impacted the homogeneity of the analysis. Moreover, each study varied widely in the optimal cutoff values for survival prediction, with the cutoff values ranging from 11 to 30 for the $ΔSUV_{max}$, from 220 to 550 mL for MTV, and from 415 to 2955 for TLG. The small number of patients have also influenced the reliability of these results.

Most recently, Kostakoglu and colleagues[61] confirmed baseline TMTV and TLG to be independent predictors of PFS and OS, in a quartile analysis, after first-line immunochemotherapy in 1334 patients with DLBCL enrolled in the phase III GOYA trial. In this study, TMTV and TLG were both found to be predictors of outcome (HR, 2.21 [95% CI, 1.48–3.29; $P < .0001$], and HR, 1.91 [95% CI, 1.28–2.85; $P = .0005$], respectively), but SUV_{max} was not a reliable predictor of outcome ($P = .38$). In COO analysis in 880 patients, better differentiation was observed in the ABC/unclassified subtypes compared with the GCB group (HR, 3.08; 95% CI, 1.49–6.37; $P = .0012$) than GCB (HR, 2.30; 95% CI, 1.05–5.01; $P = .0176$). This finding suggests that, even in this group with an unfavorable outcome, a better diagnostic group can be separated from that with a worse outcome with low MTVs, which could be used as a factor for better patient management algorithms.

In summary, although the role of MTV and TLG in HL seems to be less promising owing to the high predictive value of interim PET assessment with Lugano classification, its role in DLBCL is also not established despite promising data. If its validity is proven, it may provide a more optimal methodology to accurately predict PFS thus may better serve clinicians to design risk-adapted therapeutic strategies.

Primary Mediastinal Large B-cell Lymphoma

Primary mediastinal large B-cell lymphoma (PMBCL) is a rare subtype of DLBCL that derives from the thymic B cells. Its clinical and molecular characteristics are distinct from other subtypes of DLBCL and, in fact, closely resemble those of nodular sclerosing HL, thus, has a more favorable outcome than that of DLBCL.[62] Although there is a lack of consensus about the optimal therapeutic strategy for newly diagnosed PMCBL, highly curative strategies were developed with novel treatments such as immune checkpoint inhibitors and adoptive T-cell therapy.[62] It is important to be accurately risk stratify PMBCL patients particularly using imaging studies to initiate the best treatment strategy. After the completion of curative therapy, treatment response assessment with FDG PET/CT is challenging because of the invariably present hypermetabolic (Deauville score 4–5), residual mediastinal mass. Therefore, the quantitative evaluation of the baseline PET may be a clinically more useful test to predict response and outcome. The International Extranodal Lymphoma Study Group has investigated the value of MTVs at baseline in 103 patients with primary PMBCL who received combination chemoimmunotherapy. The MTV was estimated using a threshold method based on 25% of the SUV_{max}. These investigators found TLG to be an independent predictor of PFS ($P < .001$) and OS ($P = .001$).[63] The 5-year OS was 100% for patients with a low TLG versus 80% for those with a high TLG ($P = .0001$), and the corresponding values for PFS were 99% versus 64%, respectively (HR, 1.36; $P < .0001$). It is yet to be proven that these analyses prove superior to D-5PS and SUV_{max} with regard to predicting outcome. In another study, Pinnix and colleagues[64] retrospectively evaluated the prognostic value of MTV and TLG at baseline in a cohort of 65 patients with PMBCL who were treated with DA-R-EPOCH. At a median follow-up of 36.6 months, high MTV and TLG were associated with inferior PFS (MTV > 323.6 mL: HR, 11.5 [$P = .019$]; TLG > 3941.4: HR, 8.99 [$P = .005$]); the 2-year PFS was 67.1% versus 96.8%. On multivariable analysis, only TLG retained statistical significance ($P = .049$). A model combining baseline TLG and end-of-therapy Deauville score identified patients at increased risk of progression.

MTV determined by PET-CT is a promising prognostic indicator in PMBCL treated with standard first-line chemotherapy regimens. Further investigations with multicenter studies are necessary to establish a role for MTVs in the management scheme of PMBCL.

Follicular Lymphoma

Follicular lymphoma (FL) is a clinically and biologically heterogeneous disease with variable prognosis among individuals.[65] Although FL is associated with a long-term disease control, the disease tends to relapse. There is considerable evidence that achieving a complete metabolic response at the end of treatment is a powerful predictor of long-term survival in FL; disease progression within 2 years of initial diagnosis after first-line treatment with chemoimmunotherapy predicts a 5-year OS of approximately only 50%.[66] If high-risk patients can be objectively identified at initial staging, a survival benefit can be introduced early during the disease process, especially with the relapsing disease biology, and the inherent clinical heterogeneity of this disease. There is an unmet clinical need for identifying patients at high risk of progression in high tumor burden FL with the insufficiency of current prognostic models.

Meignan and colleagues[67] reported that the baseline MTV characteristics identify patients who would respond poorly to immunochemotherapy in a pooled centrally reviewed retrospective analysis of 185 patients with a high tumor burden FL treated in different prospective clinical trials.

Using a fixed threshold of 41% of the SUV_{max}, the median MTV was 297 cm^3 and the optimal cutoff identified was 510 cm^3, with a markedly inferior survival in patients with TMTV of greater than 510 cm^3. The 5-year PFS was 33% versus 65% (HR, 2.90; $P < .001$), and the 5-year OS was 85% versus 95% (HR, 3.45; $P = .010$). On multivariable analysis, MTV and FLIPI2 score (HR, 2.2; $P = .002$ for both) were independent predictors of PFS. In combination, they identify 3 risk groups: high MTV and intermediate to high FLIPI2 score with a 5-year PFS of 20% (HR, 5.0; $P < .001$), high TMTV or intermediate to high FLIPI2 score with 5-year PFS of 46% (HR, 2.1; $P = .007$), and low TMTV and low FLIP2 with 5-year PFS of 69%.

More recently, the same group of investigators proposed a model incorporating MTV at baseline and end of induction PET imaging results for early risk stratification in patients with high tumor burden FL.[68] In 159 patients with FL from 3 prospective trials (2 Lymphoma Study Association studies and 1 Fondazione Italiana Linfomi trial), with a median follow-up of 64 months, high TMTV (>510 cm^3) and positive end of induction PET result were independent risk factors for prediction of progression. This combination stratified the population into 3 risk groups: patients with no risk factors, patients with 1 risk factor, and patients with both risk factors had a 5-year PFS of 67% versus 33% versus 23%, respectively. The 2-year PFS were, respectively, 90% versus 61% and 46%. This model seemed to enhance the prognostic value of PET for identifying a subset of patients with a very high risk of progression and early treatment failure at 2 years.

These preliminary results warrant further validation to consider MTV as a parameter to use in various management strategies in high burden FL.

In the role of volumetric measurements in predicting outcomes, as a preliminary conclusion, MTV tends to be superior to ΔSUV_{max} in predictive values of survival, and a high MTV is significantly associated with poorer survival in patients with DLBCL treated with R-CHOP. Because of the heterogeneity of the presently published data, these results should be interpreted with caution. Additionally, because of measurement errors, the use of a strict cutoff value requires judicious application. The use of a lower and upper cutoff limit on both sides of the cutoff may be preferred.[69,70] In this area of research, although quite promising, there is a need for further analyses with future large-scale prospective studies and validation studies with standardized approach to segmentation methodologies to determine MTVs.

SUMMARY

Quantitative PET assessment with MTV and TLG seems to be a highly promising method to use for adaptive studies if externally proven valid. However, this methodology is still in an evolutionary phase and the published data are not always consistent. This may be on the basis of retrospective designs, small sample sizes translating to insufficient representation of risk and stage groups, and differences in treatments, as well as the varying methodologies used to measure MTVs. Currently, there is no consensus regarding the optimal segmentation algorithm or the quantitative index to assess the actual metabolic disease burden. Further trials investigating the prognostic and predictive values of MTV are warranted in large, standardized, homogeneous datasets for both the internal and external validation of this exciting method to prove or refute a role to improve on the prognostic value of conventional risk stratifying systems.

REFERENCES

1. Cheson BD, Fisher RI, Barrington SF, et al. Recommendations for initial evaluation, staging, and response assessment of Hodgkin and non-Hodgkin lymphoma: the Lugano classification. J Clin Oncol 2014;32:3059–68.

2. Lodge M a, Chaudhry M a, Wahl RL. Noise considerations for PET quantification using maximum and peak standardized uptake value. J Nucl Med 2012; 53:1041–7.

3. Boellaard R, Delgado-Bolton R, Oyen WJ, et al. FDG PET/CT: EANM procedure guidelines for tumour imaging: version 2.0. Eur J Nucl Med Mol Imaging 2015;42:328–54.

4. Boellaard R, Krak NC, Hoekstra OS, et al. Effects of noise, image resolution , and ROI definition on the accuracy of standard uptake values : a simulation study. J Nucl Med 2004;45:1519–27.

5. Wahl RL, Jacene H, Kasamon Y, et al. From RECIST to PERCIST: evolving Considerations for PET response criteria in solid tumors. J Nucl Med 2009; 50(Suppl 1):122S–50S.

6. Vanderhoek M, Perlman SB, Jeraj R. Impact of different standardized uptake value measures on PET-based quantification of treatment response. J Nucl Med 2013;54:1188–94.

7. Boellaard R, O'Doherty MJ, Weber WA, et al. FDG PET and PET/CT: EANM procedure guidelines for tumour PET imaging: version 1.0. Eur J Nucl Med Mol Imaging 2010;37:181–200.

8. Makris NE, Huisman MC, Kinahan PE, et al. Evaluation of strategies towards harmonization of FDG PET/CT studies in multicentre trials: comparison of

scanner validation phantoms and data analysis procedures. Eur J Nucl Med Mol Imaging 2013;40:1507–15.

9. Boellaard R. Methodological aspects of multicenter studies with quantitative PET. Methods Mol Biol 2011;727:335–49.

10. Hatt M, Cheze-Le Rest C, Aboagye EO, et al. Reproducibility of 18F-FDG and 3'-deoxy-3'-18F-fluorothymidine PET tumor volume measurements. J Nucl Med 2010;51:1368–76.

11. Cheebsumon P, Yaqub M, van Velden FH, et al. Impact of [(18)F]FDG PET imaging parameters on automatic tumour delineation: need for improved tumour delineation methodology. Eur J Nucl Med Mol Imaging 2011;38:2136–44.

12. Tylski P, Stute S, Grotus N, et al. Comparative assessment of methods for estimating tumor volume and standardized uptake value in (18)F-FDG PET. J Nucl Med 2010;51:268–76.

13. Zaidi H, El Naqa I. PET-guided delineation of radiation therapy treatment volumes: a survey of image segmentation techniques. Eur J Nucl Med Mol Imaging 2010;37:2165–87.

14. Bradley J, Thorstad WL, Mutic S, et al. Impact of FDG-PET on radiation therapy volume delineation in non-small-cell lung cancer. Int J Radiat Oncol Biol Phys 2004;59:78–86.

15. Nestle U, Weber W, Hentschel M, et al. Biological imaging in radiation therapy: role of positron emission tomography. Phys Med Biol 2009;54(1):R1-25.

16. Brambilla M, Matheoud R, Secco C, et al. Threshold segmentation for PET target volume delineation in radiation treatment planning: the role of target-to-background ratio and target size. Med Phys 2008;35:1207–13.

17. Black QC, Grills IS, Kestin LL, et al. Defining a radiotherapy target with positron emission tomography. Int J Radiat Oncol Biol Phys 2004;60:1272–82.

18. Nestle U, Kremp S, Schaefer-Schuler A, et al. Comparison of different methods for delineation of 18F-FDG PET-positive tissue for target volume definition in radiotherapy of patients with non-small cell lung cancer. J Nucl Med 2005;46:1342–8.

19. Shepherd T, Teras M, Beichel RR, et al. Comparative study with new accuracy metrics for target volume contouring in PET image guided radiation therapy'. IEEE Trans Med Imaging 2012;31:2006–24.

20. Belhassen S, Zaidi H. A novel fuzzy C-means algorithm for unsupervised heterogeneous tumor quantification in PET. Med Phys 2010;37:1309–24.

21. Chiti A, Kirienko M, Grégoire V. Clinical use of PET-CT data for radiotherapy planning: what are we looking for? Radiother Oncol 2010;96:277–9.

22. Christian P. Use of a precision fillable clinical simulator phantom for PET/CT scanner validation in multi-center clinical trials: the SNM Clinical Trials Network (CTN) Program. J Nucl Med 2012;53(suppl):437.

23. Zijlstra JM, Boellaard R, Hoekstra OS. Interim positron emission tomography scan in multi-center studies: optimization of visual and quantitative assessments. Leuk Lymphoma 2009;50:1748–9.

24. Scheuermann JS, Saffer JR, Karp JS, et al. Qualification of PET scanners for use in multicenter cancer clinical trials: the American College of Radiology Imaging Network experience. J Nucl Med 2009;50:1187–93.

25. Sunderland JJ, Christian PE. Quantitative PET/CT scanner performance characterization based upon the SNMMI clinical trial network oncology clinical simulator phantom. J Nucl Med 2015;56:145–52.

26. Kuruvilla J, Keating A, Crump M. How I treat relapsed and refractory Hodgkin lymphoma. Blood 2011;117:4208–17.

27. Gobbi PG, Ghirardelli ML, Solcia M, et al. Image-aided estimate of tumor burden in Hodgkin's disease: evidence of its primary prognostic importance. J Clin Oncol 2001;19:1388–94.

28. Gobbi PG, Broglia C, Di Giulio G, et al. The clinical value of tumor burden at diagnosis in Hodgkin lymphoma. Cancer 2004;101:1824–34.

29. Lister TA, Crowther D, Sutcliffe SB, et al. Report of a committee convened to discuss the evaluation and staging of patients with Hodgkin's disease: Cotswolds meeting. J Clin Oncol 1989;7:1630–6.

30. Hasenclever D, Diehl V. A prognostic score for advanced Hodgkin's disease: international prognostic factors project on advanced Hodgkin's disease. N Engl J Med 1998;339:1506–14.

31. Diehl V, Thomas RK, Re D. Part II: Hodgkin's lymphoma: diagnosis and treatment. Lancet Oncol 2004;5:19–26.

32. Hoppe RT, Advani RH, Bierman PJ, et al. NCCN Hodgkin disease clinical practice guidelines in oncology, 2006 v.1. Available at: http://www.nccn.org. Accessed January 6, 2006.

33. Tseng D, Rachakonda LP, Su Z, et al. Interim-treatment quantitative PET parameters predict progression and death among patients with Hodgkin's disease. Radiat Oncol 2012;7:5.

34. Ashley Knight, SNM 2014.

35. Hussien AE, Furth C, Schönberger S, et al. FDG-PET response prediction in pediatric Hodgkin's lymphoma: impact of metabolically defined tumor volumes and individualized SUV measurements on the positive predictive value. Cancers (Basel) 2015;7:287–304.

36. Song MK, Chung JS, Lee JJ, et al. Metabolic tumor volume by positron emission tomography/computed tomography as a clinical parameter to determine therapeutic modality for early stage Hodgkin's lymphoma. Cancer Sci 2013;104:1656–61.

37. Kanoun S, Rossi C, Berriolo-Riedinger A, et al. Baseline metabolic tumour volume is an independent prognostic factor in Hodgkin lymphoma. Eur J Nucl Med Mol Imaging 2014;41:1735–43.

38. Cottereau AS, Versari A, Loft A, et al. Prognostic value of baseline metabolic tumor volume in early stage Hodgkin's lymphoma in the standard arm of H10 trial. Blood 2018;131:1456–63.

39. Akhtari M, Milgrom SA, Pinnix CC, et al. Reclassifying patients with early-stage Hodgkin lymphoma based on functional radiographic markers at presentation. Blood 2018;131:84–94.

40. Kanoun S, Tal I, Berriolo-Riedinger A, et al. Influence of software tool and methodological aspects of total metabolic tumor volume calculation on baseline [18F]FDG PET to predict survival in Hodgkin lymphoma. PLoS One 2015;10(10): e0140830.

41. Moskowitz AJ, Schöder H, Gavane S. Prognostic significance of baseline metabolic tumor volume in relapsed and refractory Hodgkin lymphoma. Blood 2017;130(20):2196–203.

42. Pfreundschuh M, Ho AD, Cavallin-Stahl E, et al. Prognostic significance of maximum tumour (bulk) diameter in young adults with good-prognosis diffuse large-B-cell lymphoma treated with CHOP-like chemotherapy with or without rituximab: an exploratory analysis of the MabThera International Trial Group (MInT) study. Lancet Oncol 2008;9: 435–44.

43. Brice P, Bastion Y, Lepage E, et al. Comparison of low-tumor-burden follicular lymphomas be- tween an initial no-treatment policy, prednimustine, or interferon alfa: a randomized study from the Group d'Etude des Lymphomes Folliculares. J Clin Oncol 1997;15:1110–7.

44. Rogasch Jmm, Hundsdoerfer P, Hoffheinz F, et al. Pretherapeutic FDG PET total metabolic tumor volume predicts response to induction therapy in pediatric Hodgkin's lymphoma. BMC Cancer 2018; 18(1):521.

45. Song MK, Chung JS, Shin HJ, et al. Clinical significance of metabolic tumor volume by PET/CT in stages II and III of diffuse large B cell lymphoma without extranodal site involvement. Ann Hematol 2012;91:697–703.

46. Manohar K, Mittal BR, Bhattacharya A, et al. Prognostic value of quantitative parameters derived on initial staging 18F-fluorodeoxyglucose positron emission tomography/computed tomography in patients with high-grade non-Hodgkin's lymphoma. Nucl Med Commun 2012;33(9):974–81.

47. Sasanelli M, Meignan M, Haioun C, et al. Pretherapy metabolic tumour volume is an independent predictor of outcome in patients with diffuse large B-cell lymphoma. Eur J Nucl Med Mol Imaging 2014;41: 2017–22.

48. Kim TM, Paeng JC, Chun IK, et al. Total lesion glycolysis in positron emission tomography is a better predictor of outcome than the International Prognostic Index for patients with diffuse large B cell lymphoma. Cancer 2013;119:1195–202.

49. Kim J, Hong J, Kim SG, et al. Prognostic value of metabolic tumor volume estimated by (18)F-FDG positron emission tomography/computed tomography in patients with diffuse large B-cell lymphoma of stage II or III disease. Nucl Med Mol Imaging 2014;48:187–95.

50. Adams HJ, de Klerk JM, Fijnheer R, et al. Prognostic superiority of the National Comprehensive Cancer Network International Prognostic Index over pretreatment whole-body volumetric-metabolic FDG-PET/CT metrics in diffuse large B-cell lymphoma. Eur J Haematol 2015;94:532–9.

51. Xie M, Zhai W, Cheng S, et al. Predictive value of F-18 FDG PET/CT quantization parameters for progression-free survival in patients with diffuse large B-cell lymphoma. Hematology 2016;21(2):99–105.

52. Song MK, Chung JS, Shin HJ, et al. Prognostic value of metabolic tumor volume on PET/CT in primary gastrointestinal diffuse large B cell lymphoma. Cancer Sci 2012;103:477–82.

53. Mikhaeel NG, Smith D, Dunn JT, et al. Combination of baseline metabolic tumour volume and early response on PET/CT improves progression-free survival prediction in DLBCL. Eur J Nucl Med Mol Imaging 2016;43:1209–19.

54. Zhou M, Chen Y, Huang H, et al. Prognostic value of TLG of baseline FDG PET/CT in DLBCL. Oncotarget 2016;7:83544–53.

55. Cottereau AS, Lanic H, Mareschal S, et al. Molecular profile and FDG-PET/CT total metabolic tumor volume improve risk classification at diagnosis for patients with diffuse large B-cell lymphoma. Clin Cancer Res 2016;22:3801.

56. Xie M, Wu K, Liu Y, et al. Predictive value of F-18 FDG PET/CT quantization parameters in diffuse large B cell lymphoma: a meta-analysis with 702 participants. Med Oncol 2015;32:446.

57. Gallicchio R, Mansueto G, Simeon V, et al. 18 FDG PET/CT quantization parameters as predictors of outcome in patients with diffuse large B-cell lymphoma. Eur J Haematol 2014;92:382–9.

58. Toledano MN, Desbordes P, Banjar A, et al. Combination of baseline FDG PET/CT total metabolic tumour volume and gene expression profile have a robust predictive value in patients with diffuse large B-cell lymphoma. Eur J Nucl Med Mol Imaging 2018; 45(5):680–8.

59. Malek E, Sendilnathan A, Yellu M, et al. Metabolic tumor volume on interim PET is a better predictor of outcome in diffuse large B-cell lymphoma than semiquantitative methods. Blood Cancer J 2015; 5:e326.

60. Zhou Z, Sehn LH, Rademaker AW, et al. An enhanced International Prognostic Index (NCCN-IPI) for patients with diffuse large B-cell lymphoma treated in the rituximab era. Blood 2014;123: 837–42.

61. Kostakoglu L, Martelli M, Sehn LH, et al. Baseline PET-derived metabolic tumor volume metrics predict progression-free and overall survival in DLBCL after first-line treatment: results from the phase 3 GOYA study. Blood 2017;130:824 [abstract].

62. Dunleavy K. Primary mediastinal B-cell lymphoma: biology and evolving therapeutic strategies. Hematology Am Soc Hematol Educ Program 2017;2017: 298–303.

63. Ceriani L, Martelli M, Zinzani PL, et al. Utility of baseline 18FDG-PET/CT functional parameters in defining prognosis of primary mediastinal (thymic) large B-cell lymphoma. Blood 2015;126:950–6.

64. Pinnix CC, Ng AK, Dabaja BS, et al. Positron emission tomography-computed tomography predictors of progression after DA-R-EPOCH for PMBCL. Blood Adv 2018;2:1334–43.

65. Sutamtewagul G, Link BK. Novel treatment approaches and future perspectives in follicular lymphoma. Ther Adv Hematol 2019;10. 2040620718820510.

66. Maurer MJ, Bachy E, Ghesquieres H, et al. Early event status informs subsequent outcome in newly diagnosed follicular lymphoma. Am J Hematol 2016;91:1096–101.

67. Meignan M, Cottereau AS, Versari A, et al. Baseline metabolic tumor volume predicts outcome in high-tumor-burden follicular lymphoma: a pooled analysis of three multicenter studies. J Clin Oncol 2016;34: 3618–26.

68. Cottereau AS, Versari A, Luminari S, et al. Prognostic model for high-tumor-burden follicular lymphoma integrating baseline and end-induction PET: a LYSA/FIL study. Blood 2018; 131:2449–53.

69. Laffon E, Marthan R. On the Cutoff of Baseline Total Metabolic Tumor Volume in High-Tumor-Burden Follicular Lymphoma. J Clin Oncol 2017;35:919–20.

70. Itti E, Lin C, Dupuis J, et al. Prognostic value of interim 18F-FDG PET in patients with diffuse large B-Cell lymphoma: SUV-based assessment at 4 cycles of chemotherapy. J Nucl Med 2009;50: 527–33.

71. Park S, Moon SH, Park LC, et al. The impact of baseline and interim PET/CT parameters on clinical outcome in patients with diffuse large B cell lymphoma. Am J Hematol 2012;87(9): 937–40.

Evolving Role of PET-Based Novel Quantitative Techniques in the Management of Hematological Malignancies

William Y. Raynor, BS[a,b], Mahdi Zirakchian Zadeh, MD, MHM[c],
Esha Kothekar, MD[a], Dani P. Yellanki, BS[a],
Abass Alavi, MD, MD (Hon), PhD (Hon), DSc (Hon)[a,*]

KEYWORDS

- Quantification • Cancer • Lymphoma • Multiple myeloma • FDG • PET-CT

KEY POINTS

- FDG-PET/computed tomography can be readily applied to the assessment and monitoring of many hematological malignancies.
- Current methods of interpreting images have succeeded in identifying disease activity for the purposes of diagnosis and follow-up.
- Impaired reproducibility and ability to determine total disease activity are major limitations faced by current practices.
- The precision and accuracy of interpreting PET images can be improved with novel quantitative techniques that set objective standards and consolidate metrics of systemic disease activity measurements over generalizing data that are based on the sites of a few focal lesions.

INTRODUCTION

PET with ^{18}F-flurodeoxyglucose (FDG) exploits the increased glucose uptake by cancer cells, making FDG-PET a valuable imaging modality in various malignancies. In the domain of lymphoma, gallium-67 scintigraphy was widely used in the 1980s and 1990s in disease evaluation and monitoring but has since become replaced by FDG-PET due to the latter's superior sensitivity and specificity.[1,2] In addition, FDG-PET has the advantage of quantification of tracer uptake, which is often reported as a standardized uptake value (SUV) defined as detected activity normalized to injected dose and patient body weight. Although the maximum SUV (SUVmax) is used more commonly in clinical practice, investigations in new quantitative techniques have shown value in parameters such as the mean SUV (SUVmean) and global uptake.[3,4]

Combined PET imaging with computed tomography (CT) allows for coregistration of molecular and anatomic information, improving accuracy of PET findings by allowing metabolic activity detected by PET to be localized. PET/CT also has the advantage of using CT information for attenuation correction of PET images. Guidelines for the role of FDG-PET/CT in the diagnosis, staging, and assessment of relapse of hematological malignancies have been consolidated by organizations such as the European Society for Medical Oncology (ESMO) and International Working Group (IWG).[5,6] Since the wide acceptance of hybrid PET/CT imaging, many methods of

[a] Department of Radiology, University of Pennsylvania, 3400 Spruce Street, Philadelphia, PA 19104, USA;
[b] Drexel University College of Medicine, 2900 W Queen Lane, Philadelphia, PA 19129, USA; [c] Department of Radiology, Children's Hospital of Philadelphia, 3401 Civic Center Boulevard, Philadelphia, PA 19104, USA
* Corresponding author. 3400 Spruce Street, Philadelphia, PA 19104, USA.
E-mail address: abass.alavi@uphs.upenn.edu

PET Clin 14 (2019) 331–340
https://doi.org/10.1016/j.cpet.2019.03.003
1556-8598/19/© 2019 Elsevier Inc. All rights reserved.

segmentation and quantification still rely on mono-modal images, although new studies have investigated simultaneous joint segmentation of PET and CT images.[7–9] Novel methods of segmentation and quantification that represent total disease activity rather than focal activity may increase the utility of FDG-PET in the assessment, monitoring, and management of hematological malignancies, as these techniques are further developed and validated.

ASSESSMENT OF LYMPHOMA

Lymphoma is a group of heterogeneous lymphoid malignancy characterized by clonal proliferation of lymphocytes and is classified as either Hodgkin lymphoma (HL) or non-Hodgkin lymphoma (NHL).[10,11] FDG accumulates in activated lymphocytes, eosinophils, neutrophils, histiocytes, and plasma cells present in lymphoma and the reactive inflammatory response.[2] A 2005 study by Juweid and colleagues[12] found that FDG-PET findings combined with International Workshop Criteria (IWC) can assess response to therapy more accurately than use of IWC alone. Based on this study's findings, the IWG revised the criteria of response of NHL and HL in 2007, and FDG-PET became the standard method of evaluation for NHL and HL.[6]

A study by Pelosi and colleagues[13] compared the utility of conventional diagnostic methods (bone marrow biopsy and contrast-enhanced CT) and that of FDG-PET/CT and determined that FDG-PET/CT had a role in staging and assessment of treatment in HL and NHL. In addition, Schaefer and colleagues[14] found PET with nonenhanced CT to be more specific and more sensitive than contrast-enhanced CT in patients with HL and high-grade NHL. A report by Zeng and colleagues[15] examined a discrepancy between FDG-PET and MR imaging findings in a patient malignant lymphoma. The investigators concluded that MR imaging by itself could produce false-negative findings on diffusion-weighted images (DWI). As a result, the FDG-PET/MR imaging findings were discordant with those of MR images, showing significant uptake in the bone marrow and spleen on PET images. The false-negative MR imaging finding was attributed to presence of posttransfusion iron overload causing a decrease in signal intensity on DWI. This case emphasizes the importance of FDG-PET as an integral component of FDG-PET/MR imaging in lymphomas. A limitation of FDG-PET evaluation of lymphoma is presented by high physiologic FDG uptake in the brain, making MR imaging the preferred imaging modality in the case of suspicion of central nervous system involvement.[16]

Regarding the assessment of bone marrow involvement, FDG-PET is superior to CT because of its ability to detect early disease activity. A study noted that despite the accuracy of FDG-PET/CT in determining bone marrow involvement in newly diagnosed diffuse large B-cell lymphoma (DLBCL), it is not useful in follicular lymphoma (FL). The investigators found that when bone marrow biopsy (BMB) is used as reference standard, the sensitivity and specificity of FDG-PET/CT in detecting bone marrow involvement in DLBCL were both 100%, but in FL the sensitivity and specificity were 0% and 72.7%, respectively.[17] Because the sensitivity of FDG-PET depends on cell types involved, positive FDG-PET/CT findings may replace BMB in DLBCL, although BMB should be done in negative FDG-PET/CT in patients with advanced DLBCL to assess discordant bone marrow involvement.[17,18] In early as well as advanced stage HL, FDG-PET/CT has rendered routine BMB unnecessary.[19–24]

MONITORING LYMPHOMA

ESMO guidelines recommend interim FDG-PET in the evaluation of patients with HL.[5] Interim FDG-PET/CT is performed in patients with lymphoma after the conclusion of 1 to 4 cycles of treatment, most commonly after 2 cycles. Interim PET imaging has the advantage of showing changes in the tumor metabolic activity after the start of treatment, even before it becomes apparent structurally[25] (**Fig. 1**). This advantage is particularly important in advanced stage HL as patients might need additional radiotherapy.[26] Thus, interim FDG-PET may also prevent unnecessary overtreatment and the associated side effects. In patients who have early-stage HL, interim PET/CT can identify patients who do not require further radiotherapy and are likely to achieve complete metabolic response.[27] As with the advanced stages, interim FDG-PET/CT is used in clinical trials to select patients who require modification of treatment regimen.[2] In a study that evaluated FDG uptake according to a 5-point scale, interim PET was found to have a high negative predictive value (NPV) of 94% and a 73% positive predictive value in HL.[28]

In an effort to improve the predictive value of interim PET, a method called ΔSUVmax, which considers the changes between baseline and interim FDG uptake, has been investigated. Some studies have concluded that ΔSUVmax is a strong predictor of disease response to therapy.[29–32] In addition, metabolic tumor volume (MTV) and total lesion glycolysis (TLG) are being investigated by some groups to improve interim

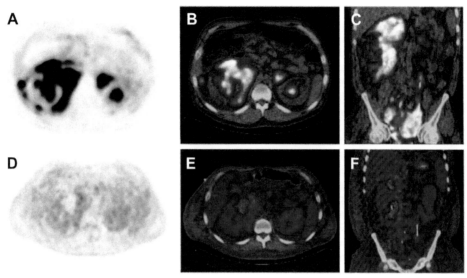

Fig. 1. Baseline (*A–C*) and interim (*D–F*) FDG-PET/CT imaging of a 40-year-old patient with Burkitt lymphoma. Diffuse abdominal adenopathy and soft tissue masses in the abdomen and pelvis show increased FDG uptake at baseline, with significant reduction in metabolic activity observed at interim after 1 cycle of rituximab contain-ing-chemotherapy. (*From* Valls L, Badve C, Avril S, et al. FDG-PET imaging in hematological malignancies. Blood Rev 2016;30(4):317–31; with permission.)

PET as an assessment tool in HL and NHL.[33–38] These parameters could be superior to SUVmax in delineating and categorizing patients based on the risk.[39] However, larger and well-designed studies are required to confirm their role.

In HL, PET/CT is more accurate at the end of treatment to assess resolution as compared with CT alone.[40] In a study, FDG-PET/CT was able to differentiate between residual active disease and fibrotic mass with a sensitivity ranging from 43% to 100% and specificity from 67% to 100%.[41] Furthermore, several studies have found a very high NPV to rule out relapse.[42,43]

The Deauville 5-point scale was developed in 2009 at the First International Workshop on PET in Deauville, France, after successful conduct of numerous trials that showed PET as a reliable tool in evaluation of staging and assessment of treatment strategies in patients with lymphoma.[44] The scale relies on uptake in the target area relative to mediastinal and hepatic SUVmax. A recent study showed that if a score of 4 and 5 is considered positive, there is a higher diagnostic accuracy in HL and NHL.[45] Alternatively, the Lugano classification for initial evaluation, staging, and response assessment for NHL and HL was formed in 2013 in Lugano, Switzerland, and is classified into 4 categories: complete metabolic response, partial metabolic response, no metabolic response, and progressive metabolic disease.[46] As new techniques are validated and malignant lesions are more readily segmented for the purpose of global

assessment, reliance on SUVmax and classifications for findings will become more obsolete.

TREATMENT ASSESSMENT IN LYMPHOMA

The treatment strategies for early-stage lymphoma have evolved over the years. Patients achieved long-term survival due to introduction of novel chemotherapies and radiotherapies. However, over the course of time, it became more apparent that therapies such as mantle-field radiotherapy and chemotherapies like mechlorethamine, vincristine, procarbazine, and prednisone (MOPP) had serious side effects. Mantle-field radiotherapy led to cardiovascular disease, hypothyroidism, and even secondary cancers.[47–50] The MOPP regimen was associated with gonadal dysfunction and secondary cancers.[51,52] Studies were conducted to establish treatment strategies to minimize side effects. The chemotherapy-radiotherapy regimen of doxorubicin, bleomycin, vinblastine, and dacarbazine (ABVD) followed by 20 Gy of involved-field radiotherapy is now a routine therapy strategy in patients with good prognosis early-stage HL. Advanced stage HL is usually treated with 6 to 8 cycles of ABVD or the more intense regimen of bleomycin, etoposide, doxorubicin, cyclophosphamide, vincristine, procarbazine, prednisolone (BEACOPPesc), and radiotherapy.

Despite development of these therapeutic strategies, there is a need for further investigation into individualizing therapy in HL. The RAPID trial was one such trial in which patients with stage IA/IIA nonbulky HL were assessed after 3 cycles of ABVD whether they required further treatment with radiotherapy.[27] Of 571 patients who underwent PET scanning, 426 patients (75%) had a negative PET scan, and were further randomized to receive either radiotherapy or no treatment. Patients who had positive PET findings received another cycle of ABVD and radiotherapy. The results for patients with negative PET findings showed that the 3-year progression-free survival (PFS) in the intention-to-treat analysis was 94.6% and 90.8% for the radiotherapy and no further treatment groups, respectively. When per-protocol analysis was done, PFS was 97.1% and 90.8% for the radiotherapy and no further treatment groups, respectively. The overall survival (OS) was 97.1% and 99.0% for the radiotherapy and no further treatment groups, respectively. This study concluded that PFS and OS of patients with early-stage HL is excellent with or without radiotherapy after 3 cycles of ABVD and that radiotherapy can be avoided in patients who have negative PET findings.

In a similar investigation, the RATHL trial used interim PET to guide therapy in advanced HL.[53] Patients with advanced HL received 2 cycles of ABVD chemotherapy, and later underwent an interim FDG-PET/CT scan. Of the 1119 patients who underwent PET/CT scanning, 937 (87.3%) had negative findings. These patients were randomly assigned to either ABVD or AVD

(omitting bleomycin) and none of them received radiotherapy. The 3-year PFS and OS rate in the ABVD group were 85.7% and 97.2%, respectively; correspondingly, they were 84.4% and 97.6%, respectively in the AVD group. However, the study noted that the toxic pulmonary side effects with AVD regimen were lower compared with the ABVD regimen.

To address underestimation of tracer uptake due to the partial volume effect, partial volume correction of SUV can be performed.[4] In addition, global assessment of disease burden has been proposed as a new method of evaluating treatment response in lymphoma.[37] In a study by Taghvaei and colleagues,[54] both TLG and partial volume-corrected TLG (pvcTLG) were used to assess treatment response in relapsed or refractory FL. A thresholding algorithm was used to quantify FDG uptake in 17 patients who received targeted radioimmunotherapy (RIT) at 3 months before and 6 months after RIT (Fig. 2). All focal malignant lesions were quantified using ROVER software (ABX GmbH, Radeberg, Germany) to determine global disease burden in each patient. Compared with TLG, pvcTLG was found to decrease more after therapy. Furthermore, patients who survived at least 3 years after RIT were observed on average to have a decreased pvcTLG after therapy, whereas those who did not survive had an increase in pvcTLG after therapy. Among the same patients, TLG decreased after therapy in both surviving and deceased

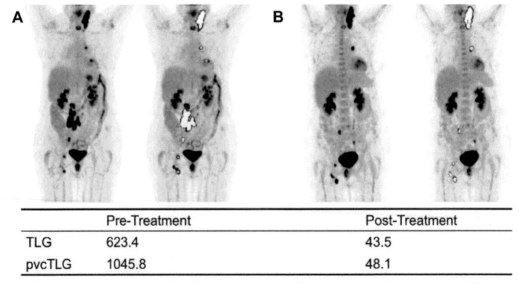

	Pre-Treatment	Post-Treatment
TLG	623.4	43.5
pvcTLG	1045.8	48.1

Fig. 2. FDG-PET images of a patient with refractory lymphoma at baseline (*A*) and after targeted RIT (*B*). Segmentation was applied using an automatic algorithm, and TLG was measured with and without partial volume correction to assess response to therapy.

patients on average, but the decrease was greater in patients who survived at least 3 years after RIT.

ROLE OF ¹⁸F-FLURODEOXYGLUCOSE-PET/ COMPUTED TOMOGRAPHY IN MULTIPLE MYELOMA

Conventional imaging techniques, such as whole-body radiograph (WBXR) and MR imaging are being challenged by increasing use of PET in multiple myeloma (MM).[55] The results of a meta-analysis that considered a total of 798 patients with MM concluded that FDG-PET/CT could detect skeletal involvement better than WBXR.[56] Other studies have suggested that FDG-PET/CT is more sensitive than MR imaging in early relapse detection.[57,58] MR imaging is also limited by slow normalization of changes in bone marrow, which could take up to a year after successful treatment.[59,60] In a study that imaged 134 patients with MM by FDG-PET/CT and MR imaging before and after 3 cycles of lenalidomide, bortezomib, and dexamethasone (RVD), 32% of patients with positive FDG-PET/CT findings at baseline had normalized findings at follow-up, whereas the rate of normalization from previously positive MR imaging assessment was 3%.[61] Presence of extramedullary disease (EMD) is a clinically important finding and may influence management of patients with MM. The sensitivity of detecting EMD by FDG-PET/CT is approximately 96%; the specificity, 78%.[62] Poorer prognoses such as shorter PFS are associated with EMD detected by FDG-PET/CT.[63]

Various PET parameters assessed at diagnosis have been observed to be predictive of prognosis. For example, a study in 192 patients with newly diagnosed MM found that presence of EMD as well as having an SUVmax greater than 4.2 were correlated with shorter PFS and shorter OS.[63] Other studies found that MTV and TLG assessed shortly after diagnosis was associated with prognosis of MM.[64,65] Dual time-point imaging (DTPI) allows for the discrimination between malignant and benign tissues by observing trends in tracer uptake after administration.[4] Data in 23 patients with MM found that change in partial volume-corrected SUVmean assessed with DTPI at baseline was a better predictor of lesion response to treatment than uncorrected SUVmean or SUVmax[66] (**Fig. 3**).

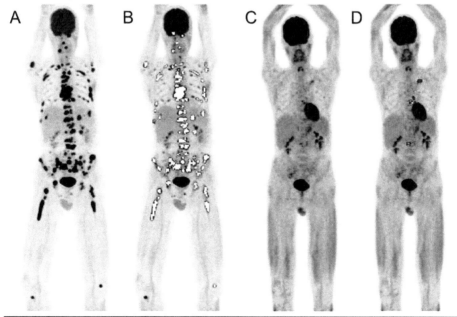

	Pre-Treatment	Post-Treatment
TLG	3359.0	12.6
pvcTLG	5280.7	19.1

Fig. 3. Baseline (*A, B*) and follow-up (*C, D*) FDG-PET images of a patient with MM before high-dose chemotherapy and 2 months after end of treatment. FDG uptake by lesions was quantified using an adaptive thresholding algorithm (ROVER software; ABX GmbH).

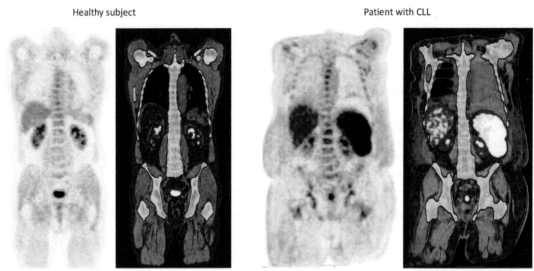

Fig. 4. FDG-PET/CT images with regions of interest used to quantify bone marrow activity in a healthy subject (*left*) and a patient with CLL (*right*). The patient with CLL presented with diffuse bone marrow FDG uptake as well as splenomegaly and Richter transformation to DLBCL. Segmentation of skeletal structures was performed based on bone Hounsfield units (OsiriX software; Pixmeo).

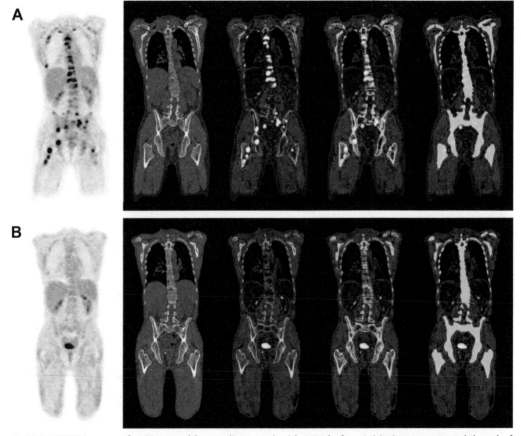

Fig. 5. FDG-PET/CT images of a 60-year-old man diagnosed with MM before initiating treatment (*A*) and after finishing the course of treatment (*B*). Segmentation of the skeleton and calculation of the global SUVmean revealed a decrease in whole bone marrow activity from 2.02 to 1.10 (OsiriX software; Pixmeo). (*From* Raynor WY, Al-Zaghal A, Zadeh MZ, et al., Metastatic seeding attacks bone marrow, not bone: rectifying ongoing misconceptions. PET Clin 2019;14(1):135–44, 141; with permission.)

Preliminary data suggest that joint PET/CT segmentation of the global bone marrow and bony skeleton is a sensitive technique in identifying disease activity in MM and smoldering myeloma (SMM).[67–71] In a prospective analysis of 39 patients with MM, 8 patients with SMM, and 24 healthy control subjects, significant differences in FDG uptake in the total bone marrow among all 3 groups were observed.[69] Some of the present authors similarly evaluated 18 patients with chronic lymphocytic leukemia (CLL) compared with 17 age-matched and sex-matched healthy subjects (**Fig. 4**). Joint segmentation was used to quantify FDG uptake in the whole bone marrow, and the results were expressed as global SUVmean. The results showed that the global SUVmean in patients with CLL was significantly higher than that of the control group (1.09 ± 0.13 vs 0.94 ± 0.19; $P = .012$), indicating that this technique may be useful in assessing related malignant conditions. In addition, NaF uptake has been measured in the axial skeleton, revealing increased systemic bone formation in MM but decreased activity in SMM compared with control subjects.[70]

Global assessment has also been applied to the assessment of therapy in MM.[72–75] High-dose chemotherapy (HDT) followed by autologous stem cell transplantation in 19 patients with MM and non–high-dose chemotherapy (non-HDT) in 9 patients were assessed by FDG-PET/CT, and significant differences between baseline and follow-up were observed in the global bone marrow of the HDT group, but not the non-HDT group (**Fig. 5**).[74] Similarly, bone metabolism assessed by NaF-PET/CT was observed to decrease in the HDT group, but not the non-HDT group.[75] Activity in the brain and spleen as assessed by global FDG uptake also has been found to change with treatment in MM, with decreased uptake in the brain and increased uptake in the spleen observed following induction treatment, HDT, and stem cell transplantation.[76,77] Thus, new segmentation techniques may play an increased role in assessing systemic effects of therapy.

SUMMARY

As the role of PET continues to grow in assessing hematological malignancies, limitations of current techniques must be addressed to best manage patients. Already, imaging with PET is able to identify sites of disease activity that are not evident on other modalities. Lesions can be accurately segmented and characterized by parameters such as TLG and SUVmean that account for volume, mean tumor activity, and partial volume correction. In addition, diffuse osseous involvement and activity in the bone marrow measured by global assessment may prove essential to the understanding of disease processes. As these new techniques are further developed and validated, popular metrics such as SUVmax will fall from common use.

REFERENCES

1. Seam P, Juweid ME, Cheson BD. The role of FDG-PET scans in patients with lymphoma. Blood 2007; 110(10):3507–16.
2. Valls L, Badve C, Avril S, et al. FDG-PET imaging in hematological malignancies. Blood Rev 2016;30(4): 317–31.
3. Raynor WY, Al-Zaghal A, Zadeh MZ, et al. Metastatic seeding attacks bone marrow, not bone: rectifying ongoing misconceptions. PET Clin 2019;14(1): 135–44.
4. Houshmand S, Salavati A, Hess S, et al. An update on novel quantitative techniques in the context of evolving whole-body PET imaging. PET Clin 2015; 10(1):45–58.
5. Dreyling M, Thieblemont C, Gallamini A, et al. ESMO consensus conferences: guidelines on malignant lymphoma. Part 2: marginal zone lymphoma, mantle cell lymphoma, peripheral T-cell lymphoma. Ann Oncol 2013;24(4):857–77.
6. Cheson BD, Pfistner B, Juweid ME, et al. Revised response criteria for malignant lymphoma. J Clin Oncol 2007;25(5):579–86.
7. Lian C, Ruan S, Denoeux T, et al. Joint tumor segmentation in PET-CT images using co-clustering and fusion based on belief functions. IEEE Trans Image Process 2019;28(2):755–66.
8. Foster B, Bagci U, Mansoor A, et al. A review on segmentation of positron emission tomography images. Comput Biol Med 2014;50:76–96.
9. Ben Bouallègue F, Tabaa YA, Kafrouni M, et al. Association between textural and morphological tumor indices on baseline PET-CT and early metabolic response on interim PET-CT in bulky malignant lymphomas. Med Phys 2017;44(9):4608–19.
10. Ansell SM. Hodgkin lymphoma: diagnosis and treatment. Mayo Clin Proc 2015;90(11):1574–83.
11. Matasar MJ, Zelenetz AD. Overview of lymphoma diagnosis and management. Radiol Clin North Am 2008;46(2):175–98, vii.
12. Juweid ME, Wiseman GA, Vose JM, et al. Response assessment of aggressive non-Hodgkin's lymphoma by integrated International Workshop Criteria and fluorine-18-fluorodeoxyglucose positron emission tomography. J Clin Oncol 2005;23(21):4652–61.
13. Pelosi E, Pregno P, Penna D, et al. Role of whole-body [18F] fluorodeoxyglucose positron emission tomography/computed tomography (FDG-PET/CT) and conventional techniques in the staging of

patients with Hodgkin and aggressive non Hodgkin lymphoma. Radiol Med 2008;113(4):578–90.

14. Schaefer NG, Hany TF, Taverna C, et al. Non-Hodgkin lymphoma and Hodgkin disease: coregistered FDG PET and CT at staging and restaging—do we need contrast-enhanced CT? Radiology 2004; 232(3):823–9.

15. Zeng F, Nogami M, Shirai T, et al. Diffusion-weighted imaging shows a false-negative finding for bone marrow involvement on 18F-FDG PET/MRI in a patient with malignant lymphoma after blood transfusion. Clin Nucl Med 2018;43(5):361–2.

16. Barrington SF, Mikhaeel NG, Kostakoglu L, et al. Role of imaging in the staging and response assessment of lymphoma: consensus of the International Conference on Malignant Lymphomas Imaging Working Group. J Clin Oncol 2014;32(27): 3048–58.

17. Teagle AR, Barton H, Charles-Edwards E, et al. Use of FDG PET/CT in identification of bone marrow involvement in diffuse large B cell lymphoma and follicular lymphoma: comparison with iliac crest bone marrow biopsy. Acta Radiol 2017;58(12): 1476–84.

18. Paone G, Itti E, Haioun C, et al. Bone marrow involvement in diffuse large B-cell lymphoma: correlation between FDG-PET uptake and type of cellular infiltrate. Eur J Nucl Med Mol Imaging 2009;36(5): 745–50.

19. Richardson SE, Sudak J, Warbey V, et al. Routine bone marrow biopsy is not necessary in the staging of patients with classical Hodgkin lymphoma in the 18F-fluoro-2-deoxyglucose positron emission tomography era. Leuk Lymphoma 2012;53(3):381–5.

20. Moulin-Romsee G, Hindié E, Cuenca X, et al. (18)F-FDG PET/CT bone/bone marrow findings in Hodgkin's lymphoma may circumvent the use of bone marrow trephine biopsy at diagnosis staging. Eur J Nucl Med Mol Imaging 2010;37(6):1095–105.

21. El-Galaly TC, d'Amore F, Mylam KJ, et al. Routine bone marrow biopsy has little or no therapeutic consequence for positron emission tomography/computed tomography-staged treatment-naive patients with Hodgkin lymphoma. J Clin Oncol 2012; 30(36):4508–14.

22. Berthet L, Cochet A, Kanoun S, et al. In newly diagnosed diffuse large B-cell lymphoma, determination of bone marrow involvement with 18F-FDG PET/CT provides better diagnostic performance and prognostic stratification than does biopsy. J Nucl Med 2013;54(8):1244–50.

23. Lim ST, Tao M, Cheung YB, et al. Can patients with early-stage diffuse large B-cell lymphoma be treated without bone marrow biopsy? Ann Oncol 2005;16(2): 215–8.

24. Adams HJ, de Klerk JM, Fijnheer R, et al. Bone marrow biopsy in diffuse large B-cell lymphoma:

useful or redundant test? Acta Oncol 2015;54(1): 67–72.

25. Römer W, Hanauske AR, Ziegler S, et al. Positron emission tomography in non-Hodgkin's lymphoma: assessment of chemotherapy with fluorodeoxyglucose. Blood 1998;91(12):4464–71.

26. Kostakoglu L, Cheson BD. State-of-the-art research on "lymphomas: role of molecular imaging for staging, prognostic evaluation, and treatment response. Front Oncol 2013;3:212.

27. Radford J, Illidge T, Counsell N, et al. Results of a trial of PET-directed therapy for early-stage Hodgkin's lymphoma. N Engl J Med 2015;372(17): 1598–607.

28. Biggi A, Gallamini A, Chauvie S, et al. International validation study for interim PET in ABVD-treated, advanced-stage Hodgkin lymphoma: interpretation criteria and concordance rate among reviewers. J Nucl Med 2013;54(5):683–90.

29. Pardal E, Coronado M, Martín A, et al. Intensification treatment based on early FDG-PET in patients with high-risk diffuse large B-cell lymphoma: a phase II GELTAMO trial. Br J Haematol 2014; 167(3):327–36.

30. Casasnovas RO, Meignan M, Berriolo-Riedinger A, et al, Groupe d'étude des lymphomes de l'adulte (GELA). SUVmax reduction improves early prognosis value of interim positron emission tomography scans in diffuse large B-cell lymphoma. Blood 2011; 118(1):37–43.

31. Nols N, Mounier N, Bouazza S, et al. Quantitative and qualitative analysis of metabolic response at interim positron emission tomography scan combined with International Prognostic Index is highly predictive of outcome in diffuse large B-cell lymphoma. Leuk Lymphoma 2014;55(4):773–80.

32. Yang DH, Ahn JS, Byun BH, et al. Interim PET/CT-based prognostic model for the treatment of diffuse large B cell lymphoma in the post-rituximab era. Ann Hematol 2013;92(4):471–9.

33. Wang H, Shen G, Jiang C, et al. Prognostic value of baseline, interim and end-of-treatment 18F-FDG PET/CT parameters in extranodal natural killer/T-cell lymphoma: a meta-analysis. PLoS One 2018; 13(3):e0194435.

34. Kim HJ, Lee R, Choi H, et al. Application of quantitative indexes of FDG PET to treatment response evaluation in indolent lymphoma. Nucl Med Mol Imaging 2018;52(5):342–9.

35. Kim TM, Paeng JC, Chun IK, et al. Total lesion glycolysis in positron emission tomography is a better predictor of outcome than the International Prognostic Index for patients with diffuse large B cell lymphoma. Cancer 2013;119(6):1195–202.

36. Basu S, Alavi A. PET-based personalized management in clinical oncology: an unavoidable path for the foreseeable future. PET Clin 2016;11(3):203–7.

37. Basu S, Zaidi H, Salavati A, et al. FDG PET/CT methodology for evaluation of treatment response in lymphoma: from "graded visual analysis" and "semiquantitative SUVmax" to global disease burden assessment. Eur J Nucl Med Mol Imaging 2014; 41(11):2158–60.

38. Berkowitz A, Basu S, Srinivas S, et al. Determination of whole-body metabolic burden as a quantitative measure of disease activity in lymphoma: a novel approach with fluorodeoxyglucose-PET. Nucl Med Commun 2008;29(6):521–6.

39. Cheson BD, Kostakoglu L. FDG-PET for early response assessment in lymphomas: part 2—diffuse large B-cell lymphoma, use of quantitative PET evaluation. Oncology (Williston Park) 2017;31(1):71–6.

40. Cerci JJ, Trindade E, Pracchia LF, et al. Cost effectiveness of positron emission tomography in patients with Hodgkin's lymphoma in unconfirmed complete remission or partial remission after first-line therapy. J Clin Oncol 2010;28(8):1415–21.

41. Terasawa T, Nihashi T, Hotta T, et al. 18F-FDG PET for posttherapy assessment of Hodgkin's disease and aggressive Non-Hodgkin's lymphoma: a systematic review. J Nucl Med 2008;49(1):13–21.

42. Panizo C, Pérez-Salazar M, Bendandi M, et al. Positron emission tomography using 18F-fluorodeoxyglucose for the evaluation of residual Hodgkin's disease mediastinal masses. Leuk Lymphoma 2004;45(9):1829–33.

43. Weihrauch MR, Re D, Scheidhauer K, et al. Thoracic positron emission tomography using 18F-fluorodeoxyglucose for the evaluation of residual mediastinal Hodgkin disease. Blood 2001;98(10):2930–4.

44. Meignan M, Gallamini A, Meignan M, et al. Report on the first International Workshop on interim-PET-scan in lymphoma. Leuk Lymphoma 2009;50(8):1257–60.

45. Fallanca F, Alongi P, Incerti E, et al. Diagnostic accuracy of FDG PET/CT for clinical evaluation at the end of treatment of HL and NHL: a comparison of the Deauville criteria (DC) and the International Harmonization Project Criteria (IHPC). Eur J Nucl Med Mol Imaging 2016;43(10):1837–48.

46. Cheson BD, Fisher RI, Barrington SF, et al. Recommendations for initial evaluation, staging, and response assessment of Hodgkin and non-Hodgkin lymphoma: the Lugano classification. J Clin Oncol 2014;32(27):3059–68.

47. Travis LB, Gospodarowicz M, Curtis RE, et al. Lung cancer following chemotherapy and radiotherapy for Hodgkin's disease. J Natl Cancer Inst 2002;94(3): 182–92.

48. Deniz K, O'Mahony S, Ross G, et al. Breast cancer in women after treatment for Hodgkin's disease. Lancet Oncol 2003;4(4):207–14.

49. Hancock SL, Cox RS, McDougall IR. Thyroid diseases after treatment of Hodgkin's disease. N Engl J Med 1991;325(9):599–605.

50. Swerdlow AJ, Higgins CD, Smith P, et al. Myocardial infarction mortality risk after treatment for Hodgkin disease: a collaborative British cohort study. J Natl Cancer Inst 2007;99(3):206–14.

51. Boivin JF, Hutchison GB, Zauber AG, et al. Incidence of second cancers in patients treated for Hodgkin's disease. J Natl Cancer Inst 1995;87(10): 732–41.

52. van der Kaaij MA, Heutte N, Meijnders P, et al. Premature ovarian failure and fertility in long-term survivors of Hodgkin's lymphoma: a European Organisation for Research and Treatment of Cancer Lymphoma Group and Groupe d'Etude des Lymphomes de l'Adulte Cohort Study. J Clin Oncol 2012;30(3):291–9.

53. Johnson P, Federico M, Kirkwood A, et al. Adapted treatment guided by interim PET-CT scan in advanced Hodgkin's lymphoma. N Engl J Med 2016;374(25):2419–29.

54. Taghvaei R, Pourhassan Shamchi S, Khosravi M, et al. Evolving role of global disease burden assessment by novel quantitative technique in patients with lymphoma following therapeutic intervention. J Nucl Med 2017;58(supplement 1):570.

55. Taghvaei R, Zirakchian Zadeh M, Østergaard B, et al. PET imaging in hematological malignancies. J Nucl Med 2017;58(supplement 1):1008.

56. van Lammeren-Venema D, Regelink JC, Riphagen II, et al. ^{18}F-fluoro-deoxyglucose positron emission tomography in assessment of myeloma-related bone disease: a systematic review. Cancer 2012;118(8): 1971–81.

57. Derlin T, Weber C, Habermann CR, et al. 18F-FDG PET/CT for detection and localization of residual or recurrent disease in patients with multiple myeloma after stem cell transplantation. Eur J Nucl Med Mol Imaging 2012;39(3):493–500.

58. Spinnato P, Bazzocchi A, Brioli A, et al. Contrast enhanced MRI and ^{18}F-FDG PET-CT in the assessment of multiple myeloma: a comparison of results in different phases of the disease. Eur J Radiol 2012;81(12):4013–8.

59. Healy CF, Murray JG, Eustace SJ, et al. Multiple myeloma: a review of imaging features and radiological techniques. Bone Marrow Res 2011;2011: 583439.

60. Walker R, Barlogie B, Haessler J, et al. Magnetic resonance imaging in multiple myeloma: diagnostic and clinical implications. J Clin Oncol 2007;25(9):1121–8.

61. Moreau P, Attal M, Caillot D, et al. Prospective evaluation of magnetic resonance imaging and [^{18}F]fluorodeoxyglucose positron emission tomography-computed tomography at diagnosis and before maintenance therapy in symptomatic patients with multiple myeloma included in the IFM/DFCI 2009 trial: results of the IMAJEM study. J Clin Oncol 2017;35(25):2911–8.

62. Lu YY, Chen JH, Lin WY, et al. FDG PET or PET/CT for detecting intramedullary and extramedullary lesions in multiple myeloma: a systematic review and meta-analysis. Clin Nucl Med 2012;37(9):833–7.

63. Zamagni E, Patriarca F, Nanni C, et al. Prognostic relevance of 18-F FDG PET/CT in newly diagnosed multiple myeloma patients treated with up-front autologous transplantation. Blood 2011;118(23): 5989–95.

64. McDonald JE, Kessler MM, Gardner MW, et al. Assessment of total lesion glycolysis by ^{18}F FDG PET/CT significantly improves prognostic value of GEP and ISS in myeloma. Clin Cancer Res 2017; 23(8):1981–7.

65. Fonti R, Larobina M, Del Vecchio S, et al. Metabolic tumor volume assessed by 18F-FDG PET/CT for the prediction of outcome in patients with multiple myeloma. J Nucl Med 2012;53(12):1829–35.

66. Taghvaei R, Østergaard B, Zirakchian Zadeh M, et al. Correlation of dual time point FDG-PET with response to chemotherapy in multiple myeloma. J Nucl Med 2017;58(supplement 1):188.

67. Zirakchian Zadeh M, Østergaard B, Raynor W, et al. Quantification of the total bone marrow activity with FDG-PET in multiple myeloma before and after treatment: comparison with a control group. J Nucl Med 2017;58(supplement 1):190.

68. Zirakchian Zadeh M, Østergaard B, Raynor W, et al. Comparison of global uptake of NaF-PET/CT in whole-body bone in multiple myeloma and healthy controls. J Nucl Med 2017;58(supplement 1):768.

69. Raynor W, Zirakchian Zadeh M, Acosta-Montenegro O, et al. Measuring bone marrow activity with FDG-PET in multiple myeloma, smoldering myeloma, and healthy subjects. J Nucl Med 2018;59(supplement 1):1420.

70. Raynor W, Zirakchian Zadeh M, Acosta-Montenegro O, et al. Systemic bone remodeling in multiple myeloma, smoldering myeloma, and healthy subjects: global assessment with NaF-PET. J Nucl Med 2018; 59(supplement 1):24.

71. Acosta-Montenegro O, Raynor W, Ayubcha C, et al. Global assessment of PET tracer uptake in the skeleton using CT segmentation: a novel approach to quantification of disease activity and whole body metabolism. J Nucl Med 2017;58(supplement 1): 1017.

72. Acosta-Montenegro O, Raynor W, Østergaard B, et al. Feasibility of using global FDG uptake in bone marrow to assess treatment of multiple myeloma. J Nucl Med 2017;58(supplement 1):189.

73. Raynor W, Acosta-Montenegro O, Østergaard B, et al. Global quantification of NaF in the skeleton: assessing bone formation in multiple myeloma patients before and after treatment. J Nucl Med 2017; 58(supplement 1):1214.

74. Zirakchian Zadeh M, Raynor W, Østergaard B, et al. Changes in bone marrow FDG uptake in multiple myeloma patients before and after treatment. J Nucl Med 2018;59(supplement 1):1430.

75. Zirakchian Zadeh M, Raynor W, Østergaard B, et al. Assessment of bone turnover in multiple myeloma patients before and after treatment. J Nucl Med 2018;59(supplement 1):1429.

76. Pourhassan Shamchi S, Østergaard B, Khosravi M, et al. Effects of chemotherapy on brain glucose metabolism in patients with multiple myeloma. J Nucl Med 2017;58(supplement 1):1262.

77. Nguyen D, Al-Zaghal A, Saboury B, et al. Quantifying metabolic activity of the spleen in patient with multiple myeloma using 18F-FDG PET/CT: comparison to normal subject and evaluation of the effect of the high-dose chemotherapy. J Nucl Med 2018; 59(supplement 1):1431.

Evolving Roles of Fluorodeoxyglucose and Sodium Fluoride in Assessment of Multiple Myeloma Patients

Introducing a Novel Method of PET Quantification to Overcome Shortcomings of the Existing Approaches

Mahdi Zirakchian Zadeh, MD, MHM[a,b],
William Y. Raynor, BS[a,c],
Siavash Mehdizadeh Seraj, MD, MHM[a], Cyrus Ayubcha, BA[a],
Esha Kothekar, MD[a], Thomas Werner, MSc[a],
Abass Alavi, MD, MD (Hon), PhD (Hon), DSc (Hon)[a,*]

KEYWORDS

- Multiple myeloma • FDG • NaF • PET/CT • Global assessment • GSUVmean
- Dual time point imaging • Atherosclerosis

KEY POINTS

- The routine use of PET/CT in patients with MM is still hampered mainly by the lack of standardized imaging criteria, resulting in poor interobserver and intraobserver reproducibility for interpretation of PET images.
- We believe the semiautomated method of quantification, GSUVmean, is able to overcome such deficiencies regarding the poor reproducibility of PET quantification in this hematologic cancer.
- Moreover, our preliminary results in evaluating the NaF uptake in thoracic aorta determined a significant difference between the average SUVmean between the myeloma patients and healthy-control subjects. This shows that NaF-PET/CT is a valuable modality in the detection of atherosclerosis at earlier stages in patients with MM.

Multiple myeloma (MM) is a malignant disorder that affects clonal proliferation of plasma cells in bone marrow and is the second most common hematologic malignancy in the United States after non-Hodgkin lymphoma.[1] Patients typically present with bone marrow infiltration of malignant plasma cells and appearance of monoclonal protein (also known as M protein) in the serum and/or urine.[2] The clinical features of the disease include hypercalcemia; renal failure; anemia; and myeloma bone diseases, such as osteolytic lesions, pathologic fractures, and osteoporosis.[3] Despite improvements in the survival rate over the years, the prognosis of patients with MM still remains poor.[4]

Osteolytic lesions are the hallmark of MM, occurring in almost all patients during the course of the disease.[5] These patients present with an imbalanced metabolism with increased osteoclastic

[a] Department of Radiology, University of Pennsylvania, 3400 Spruce Street, Philadelphia, PA 19104, USA; [b] Department of Radiology, Children's Hospital of Philadelphia, 3401 Civic Center Boulevard, Philadelphia, PA 19104, USA; [c] Drexel University College of Medicine, 2900 West Queen Lane, Philadelphia, PA 19129, USA
* Corresponding author.
E-mail address: abass.alavi@uphs.upenn.edu

PET Clin 14 (2019) 341–352
https://doi.org/10.1016/j.cpet.2019.03.004
1556-8598/19/© 2019 Elsevier Inc. All rights reserved.

and decreased osteoblastic activities, which results in osteolytic lesions.[6–8] For decades, the gold standard imaging modality for identifying lytic lesions has been based on whole-body x-ray (WBXR) radiography.[9,10] By now, it is well established that the sensitivity of plain radiographs for detecting lytic lesions is limited, because the lesions are undetectable until the bone mass is destroyed by at least 30% to 50%.[11] Therefore, the use of advanced and sensitive imaging modalities, such as PET, is necessary for early detection of osteolytic lesions.

Among PET radiotracers, the role of fluorodeoxyglucose (FDG) has been explored in characterizing MM lesions in the red marrow with high levels of sensitivity and specificity (**Fig. 1**).[12] Moreover, emerging data have shown that FDG PET/computed tomography (CT) has an important role in the prediction of outcome, evaluation of response to treatment, and the overall management of patients with MM. In addition to FDG, in recent years, the potential role of a bone-seeking PET radiopharmaceutical, ^{18}F-sodium fluoride (NaF), has been investigated for assessing loss of bone and its consequences in patients with MM. NaF is a biomarker of bone remodeling with a high level of sensitivity and reliability, and as such, has been generally used in examining a wide spectrum of skeletal disorders.[13,14] The biochemical basis for the uptake of NaF in the bone is caused by the exchange of the fluorine ion that occurs between NaF and hydroxyapatite, which results in formation of fluoroapatite.[15,16] Therefore, tracer uptake with this compound reflects regional osteoblastic activity and bone turnover.[17] In addition to evaluating osseous lesions, NaF uptake is noted in active calcification in soft

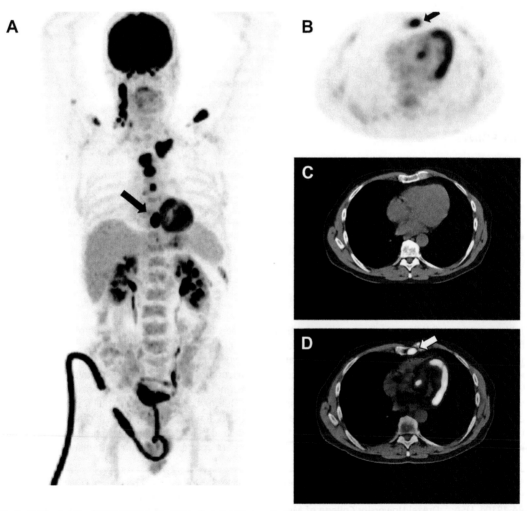

Fig. 1. Critical role of FDG PET in assessing skeletal disease in MM. A 60-year-old man newly diagnosed with MM. FDG PET revealed cervical lymphadenopathies and multiple active lesions with variable FDG uptakes in the skeleton (*A*). An active lesion in the sternum (*arrows*) was detected on PET and PET/CT (*A, B, D*) but not on CT alone (*C*).

tissues in various organs and structures including arterial atherosclerosis.

Although PET/CT has been increasingly used for assessing patients with MM over the past decade, its routine application is still hindered by several factors. According to the International Myeloma Working Group (IMWG), the main drawback of FDG PET/CT is the lack of standardized image assessment criteria, resulting in poor interobserver and intraobserver reproducibility for interpreting PET results. Therefore, to establish a defendable role for PET in MM similar to that in solid tumors and lymphomas, the development of well-defined image acquisition protocols is necessary in the near future.[18–21] We believe global disease assessment is a new method of PET quantification that can overcome the existing deficiencies and improve accuracy and reproducibility of PET findings. This quantification technique can be applied to FDG and NaF images by providing a means of evaluating the whole bone marrow and osseous structures, respectively.

In this review article, we review the available data regarding the use of FDG and NaF PET/CT in patients with MM. Then, we explore two new aspects of PET imaging for the evaluation of patients with MM: dual time point FDG-PET imaging and overall disease assessment in the red marrow and skeletal structures. We introduce the global assessment approach as a novel method of PET quantification in myeloma disease. We believe this novel method of PET quantification is able to overcome some shortcomings regarding poor reproducibility of PET measurements in this malignancy. Finally, we discuss the role of NaF in detecting atherosclerosis in the early stages of the disease.

ASSESSMENT OF OSTEOLYTIC LESIONS AND BONE MARROW INVOLVEMENT

In past years, WBXR had been accepted as the gold standard for the assessment of skeletal involvement in MM. The main shortcoming of plain radiographs is its low sensitivity of 30% to 50%, and this results in delayed diagnosis of bone destruction and staging of patients with MM.[22,23] Therefore, IMWG has recommended integrating novel imaging modalities into the evaluation of myeloma lytic lesions because of their higher sensitivity and potency in identifying bone destruction at an earlier stage than those of plain radiographs. Multiple studies have demonstrated the efficacy of FDG PET/CT as part of the workup for detecting lytic lesions, with a high sensitivity and specificity range of 80% to 100%.[24–33] For instance, Bredella and colleagues[33] showed a sensitivity of 85% and specificity of 92% for FDG PET/CT in detecting lytic lesions. In another study by Nanni and colleagues[28] on newly diagnosed patients with MM, in 16 of 28 patients with MM, additional lesions were detected by FDG PET/CT compared with WBXR. In another PET-based prospective study, 46 newly diagnosed patients with MM were evaluated. The results showed that FDG PET was superior imaging modality for identifying active lesions in 46% of patients, whereas WBXR demonstrated a better sensitivity in only 8% of the subjects examined.[25] A recent comparison between WBXR and FDG PET showed that in six of seven studies FDG PET detected more lesions at staging than conventional techniques.[24] A systematic review of 32 studies that was published in 2013 by Regelink and colleagues[34] found that compared with WBXR, MR imaging, CT, and PET/CT had significantly higher detection rates for MM-related lytic lesions. In one study comparing FDG PET/CT with WBXR and MR imaging of the spine and pelvis, it was determined that FDG PET/CT is superior to WBXR for identifying lytic lesions, whereas MR imaging was more sensitive in detecting diffuse infiltration of plasma cell in bone marrow.[25] However, the comparatively smaller MR imaging field of view represented a limitation, with a third of patients having osseous abnormalities visualized by FDG PET/CT at sites not imaged by MR imaging.[25] Another study found that FDG PET/CT and MR imaging modalities were equivalently effective in detecting focal lesions in the spine.[35] In general, based on what is well established, MR imaging is sensitive but nonspecific in many settings including those related to red marrow disorders. Therefore, the role of MR imaging in assessing hematologic malignancies is uncertain at this time.

In studies that compared the utility of FDG and NaF in MM, most authors concluded that FDG is superior to NaF for detecting osteolytic lesions (Fig. 2). For instance, in a prospective study, whole-body FDG PET/CT was positive for 343 lesions, whereas NaF PET/CT showed only 135 lytic lesions.[36] In another study in 26 patients with MM, the authors determined that NaF PET/CT scan was not of clinical value in assessing bone lesions in MM compared with FDG.[37] Despite this conclusion, the authors noted that NaF demonstrated 135 additional bone lesions, including rib fractures and degenerative changes.[37] However, in one study, some bone lesions were reported to have more intense uptake on imaging with NaF compared with FDG uptake. The authors concluded that small lytic lesions might therefore be overlooked by FDG PET/CT, representing a potential use for NaF PET/CT as

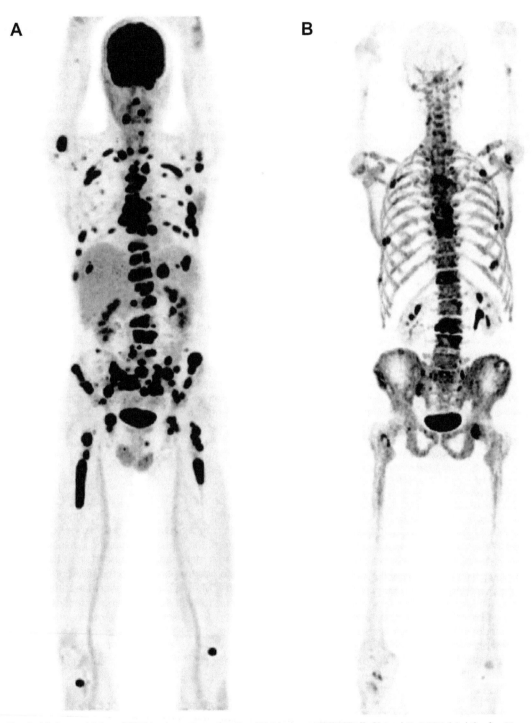

Fig. 2. High sensitivity of FDG in detection of active MM lesions. FDG PET (*left*) and NaF PET (*right*) of a 60-year-old man diagnosed with MM. The whole-body FDG PET shows numerous active lesions in the skeleton and extra-medullary sites (*A*). Whole-body NaF PET did not visualize most of the lesions detected by FDG PET (*B*).

a means of increasing sensitivity.[38] Because these patients suffer from osteolytic and osteoblastic (seen in fractures) lesions, the balance of uptake of NaF cannot differentiate between these two ongoing biologic processes. Therefore, care must be taken during accurate interpretation of the results from NaF PET/CT imaging in this population.

Previous studies have found that FDG PET/CT has the ability to determine the degree of malignant plasma cell infiltration in bone marrow.[27] For instance, in a study that correlated FDG uptake and the percentage of plasma cell in bone marrow, a negative FDG PET/CT result was associated with lowest bone marrow involvement, whereas mixed focal or diffuse pattern of FDG uptake was noted to relate to the highest rates of malignant plasma cell infiltration.[27] In another study, Ak and Gulbas[39] found a significant correlation between FDG uptake and percentage of CD38/CD138-positive myeloma cells. The authors concluded that imaging with FDG may be valuable for evaluating the degree of activity of myeloma cells in bone marrow.[39]

Overall, the intended management of patients with MM seems to be heavily influenced by FDG PET/CT findings, based on a large study in patients with 18 different types of cancer.[40] This research indicated that PET findings had the greatest impact, with 49% of cases having changes in management decisions and 42% of cases changing intended management from no treatment to treatment.[40]

PREDICTION OF PROGNOSIS

FDG PET/CT can assess prognosis of patients with newly diagnosed and relapsed or refractory MM.[41–47] Baseline findings of three focal lesions on FDG-PET/CT imaging has been correlated with poorer prognoses, such as high-risk genetic profiles, decreased progression-free survival (PFS) and overall survival (OS), and adverse changes in biomarkers, such as increased C-reactive protein, lactate dehydrogenase, and β-2 microglobulin levels.[12]

Patients Undergoing Allogeneic Stem Cell Transplant

Prediction of patient prognosis in newly diagnosed MM is enhanced by performing FDG PET/CT imaging performed before stem cell transplant. For instance, in a research project, an FDG PET/CT scan was performed in patients with MM within 30 days before allogeneic stem cell transplant. In this study, positive results were found in 32 (59%) patients, with extramedullary involvement in six (11%) patients, and an SUV_{max} of more than 4.2 in 21 (39%) patients. Extramedullary disease (EMD) and a high SUV_{max} were associated with inferior OS and PFS.[46] With a similar approach, Zamagni and colleagues[41] used FDG-PET/CT as a tool in prognostication in 192 newly diagnosed patients with MM at diagnosis and at the end of thalidomide-dexamethasone induction therapy and transplantation. They found pretreatment existence of at least three focal lesions, SUV_{max} higher than 4.2, and extramedullary involvement were associated with inferior PFS (≥3 focal lesions, 50%; SUV >4.2, 43%; EMD, 28%). SUV_{max} higher than 4.2 and involvement of extramedullary sites were also associated with inferior OS (4-year rates: 77% and 66%, respectively).

Patients with Relapsed or Progressive Disease

According to IMWG, there is a need for future investigations in relapsed and refractory MM in patients who have undergone autologous stem-cell transplantation (ASCT) and those who are not eligible for ASCT. Negative FDG PET/CT findings were predictive of a favorable prognosis in patients with relapse or progression after a previous ASCT or allogeneic stem cell transplant. However, positive FDG-PET/CT showing EMD and increased number of focal lesions predicted worse outcome including short interval time to progression and poor OS.[47]

VALUE OF FLUORODEOXYGLUCOSE PET/COMPUTED TOMOGRAPHY IN THERAPY ASSESSMENT

Assessment of therapy response represents a major domain where FDG PET/CT may prove to be more useful than conventional imaging modalities. By characterizing the metabolic activity at sites of clonal plasma cell proliferation, FDG PET/CT can accurately evaluate and monitor changes quantitatively in cancer cell activity after treatment.[35,41,42,48–51] Additionally, negative FDG PET/CT findings correlate well with a strong response to therapy.[41]

Baseline Parameters of Fluorodeoxyglucose-PET

In a study, FDG PET/CT imaging was performed in patients with MM either on the seventh day after induction treatment or before the first ASCT. It was observed that the patients who had continued presence of more than three focal lesions by the seventh day, had inferior PFS and OS, particularly in those with high-risk gene expression profiles.[48] Similarly, a significantly improved PFS and OS were observed in cases with complete suppression of FDG avidity in focal lesions before ASCT. In addition, it was shown that FDG PET/CT scans were able to predict complete response, in some cases, nearly 18 months before the findings on MR imaging or other structural imaging modalities.[48] In another investigation, persistent high tumor metabolism portrayed by FDG uptake after induction treatment correlated well with inferior PFS after ASCT; lower uptake of FDG after ASCT was also associated with greater disease suppression and prolonged OS.[41] In another study involving 239 patients who underwent neoadjuvant therapy followed by ASCT, inferior OS and event-free survival was observed in patient with more than three focal lesions on baseline FDG PET scan. Specifically, 87% of patients with three or fewer FDG-avid lesions were observed with 30-month event-free survival, whereas only 66% of patients with more than three FDG-avid lesions survived event-free in the same time. Moreover, increased overall and event-free survival was seen in patients who showed complete normalization of FDG PET uptake before stem cell transplant.[42] A study of 19 patients by Dimitrakopoulou-Strauss and colleagues[49] revealed that PFS after chemotherapy could be accurately predicted by using baseline SUV_{max}, but changes in SUV_{max} after chemotherapy were not found to correlate with PFS.

Post–Autologous Stem Cell Transplantation Assessment

A negative post-therapy PET/CT scan has been proven to be predictive of nonrelapse and a long-term disease-free survival time, whereas high post-treatment SUVs were correlated with shorter times until relapse.[52] For instance, Zamagni and colleagues[41] showed that continued FDG avidity 3 months after ASCT predicted shorter PFS. For patients determined to be PET-negative, estimates of 4-year PFS and OS were 47% and 79%, respectively, whereas for patients determined to be PET-positive, estimates of 4-year PFS and OS were 32% and 66%, respectively.[41]

Comparison Between PET and MR Imaging for Evaluation of Response to Treatment

In patients with complete or significant partial response to treatment, FDG-PET/CT showed faster normalization as compared with contrast-enhanced MR imaging. In one analysis, PET/CT helped correctly identify 16 of 20 patients (80%) who presented positive responses to treatment as compared with only 12 of 20 patients (60%) identified by MR imaging.[53] In another study, Spinnato and colleagues[32] studied 40 patients with MM and showed that in 27 patients (67.5%) with good or complete response to therapy, the normalization of findings was faster in PET-CT than in MR imaging.[32]

DETECTION OF MINIMAL RESIDUAL DISEASE IN MULTIPLE MYELOMA

Interest in evaluation and monitoring of minimal residual disease (MRD) has grown with recent advances and introduction of new drugs that have improved efficacy in the treatment of MM.[54] Cellular and molecular approaches, such as flow cytometry immunophenotyping, allele-specific oligonucleotide-polymerase chain reaction or multiplex polymerase chain reaction followed by high-throughput next-generation sequencing, have been used in the assessment of MRD. Unfortunately, these approaches have resulted in a higher number of false-negatives because of the heterogeneous pattern of bone marrow infiltration in MM.[12] Therefore, IMWG has recommended that both sensitive bone marrow-based assays be used alongside functional imaging techniques capable of detecting MRD outside the bone marrow.[12] Combining techniques allows determining whether tumor clones have been completely eradicated. In this context, FDG PET/CT has provided a great tool for assessing tumor activity and tumors' metabolic responses to given therapies. Multiple studies including a comprehensive meta-analysis showed that in complete responses after an ASCT, negative FDG PET-CT served as a robust predictor of better outcomes compared with markers of persistent metabolic activity.[35,41,55] A retrospective study assessed FDG PET/CT scans in ASCT-eligible and ASCT-ineligible patients at baseline and after treatment. Although 100 (53%) of 189 patients achieved complete response, the FDG PET/CT images were still positive in 29 (29%) of the 100 cases.[45] PFS and OS were significantly inferior in comparison with other patients (median PFS, 44 vs 84 months [P = .0009]; OS at 5 years, 70% vs 90% [P = .003]) in patients with continued FDG uptake. In addition, multivariate analysis showed that negative FDG PET/CT is a predictor of prolonged PFS and OS after treatment.[45] In another study, negative FDG PET/CT findings was associated with higher PFS and OS in patients who achieved excellent partial response after ASCT.[50]

DUAL TIME POINT IMAGING IN PATIENTS WITH MULTIPLE MYELOMA

FDG uptake in malignant tumors has been shown to consistently increase from 1-hour to 4-hour scans, whereas benign lesions and normal tissue demonstrate a decline in uptake from 1-hour to 4-hours after FDG administration.[56] As such, delayed imaging allows detection of malignant lesions with higher sensitivity and specificity compared with single time point imaging at 60 minutes.[57–59] Therefore, dual time point imaging (DTPI) has been shown to be a promising method in determining whether a lesion is malignant or benign.[59,60] However, the role of DTPI in assessing MM lesions is poorly defined in the literature. Taghvaei and colleagues[61] measured FDG uptake at 1 hour and 3 hours in patients with MM and analyzed the change in uptake over this time period using novel software (ROVER, ABX, Radeberg, Germany). The study noted that lesions with a significantly higher increase in SUVmean and partial volume corrected SUVmean were associated with partial response compared with complete response in those with stable measurements. The study concluded that DTPI with early and delayed scans could be a predictor of the degree of aggressiveness and response to chemotherapy in patients with MM (**Fig. 3**).[61]

NOVEL METHOD OF PET/COMPUTED TOMOGRAPHY QUANTIFICATION

Currently, quantification of active lesions on PET is based on assigning small regions of interest to sites of focal tracer uptake at baseline and after treatment. Because of the partial volume effect, small regions of interest result in underestimating

tracer uptake and therefore, inaccurate assessment of the actual levels of metabolic activity of the lesions examined.[62] In addition, these conventional methods are not able to show the burden of disease in the entire body because they just focus on examining a few focal lesions. Finally, the lack of a definitive standard for assigning regions of interest in patients with MM results in suboptimal reproducibility of attempted measurements. According to IMWG, lack of reproducibility and high variability among the interpreters of FDG PET/CT images are major limitations in implementing this modality in clinical practice of patients with MM. Investigators at the University of Pennsylvania and the University of Southern Denmark have described a new method for quantifying FDG uptake in the bone marrow of patients with MM, aiming to address the previously mentioned shortcomings of current quantitative techniques for assessing the degree of disease activity in the whole bone marrow of patients with MM. These investigators describe FDG PET/CT data in 39 patients with MM and eight patients with smoldering myeloma (SMM) who were examined prospectively. They compared the results from 24 healthy control subjects who were matched to patients with MM by sex and age ($\pm$5 years).[63] CT segmentation was used to measure FDG uptake on a

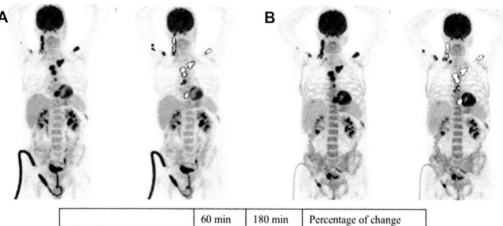

	60 min	180 min	Percentage of change
SUVmean (CR Lesions)	5.95	7.29	22.52%
SUVmean (PR Lesions)	5.58	6.98	25.08%
pvcSUVmean (CR lesions)	9.04	11.28	24.77%
pvcSUVmean (PR lesions)	8.55	11.42	33.56%

Fig. 3. Dual time point imaging to assess aggressiveness of MM lesions. FDG PET/CT scans of a 60-year-old man with newly diagnosed MM. (*A*) Pretreatment FDG PET scan 1 hour after injection of FDG tracer. (*B*) Pretreatment FDG PET scan 3 hours after injection of FDG as assessed by a novel segmentation technique (ROVER, ABX, Radeberg, Germany). The table shows the percentage of changes in the SUV$_{mean}$ and partial volume corrected (pvc) SUV$_{mean}$ of the lesions with complete response (CR) and partial response (PR) from 1-hour to 3-hour scans. (*From* Raynor WY, Al-Zaghal A, Zadeh MZ, et al. Metastatic seeding attacks bone marrow, not bone: rectifying ongoing misconceptions. PET Clin. 2019;14:135–44. https://doi.org/10.1016/j.cpet.2018.08.005; with permission.)

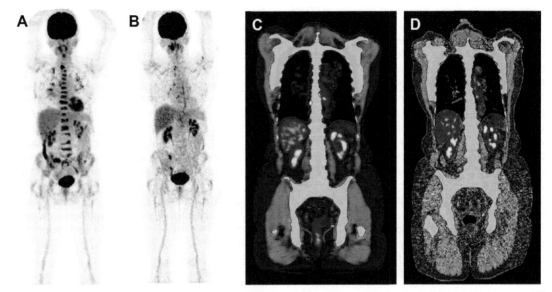

Fig. 4. Potential role of global disease assessment by PET in MM. FDG uptake changes of MM lesions before (*A*) and after the treatment (*B*). High diffuse FDG uptake is observed in the entire spine before the treatment (*A*), whereas substantial reduction in FDG uptake is visually noted after the treatment (*B*). Segmentation of the entire skeleton followed by a closing algorithm allows for one to perform global disease assessment (OsiriX software, Pixmeo SARL, Bernex, Switzerland) (*C, D*). The pretreatment global average SUVmean (*C*) was 3.1 and decreased to 1.8 after the completion of the treatment (*D*).

fused PET/CT image. The measured global SUV-mean for MM, SMM, and control subjects were 1.71 ± 0.49, 1.27 ± 0.15, and 1.11 ± 0.19, respectively. Because GSUVmean showed a significant difference among the different groups, this technique seems to reflect the degree of disease activity present in subjects with myeloma caused by

bone marrow infiltration by malignant cells.[63] In addition, changes in the whole bone marrow uptake of FDG before and after treatment were assessed with this method in 19 patients with MM scheduled for treatment with high dose treatment (HDT) followed by ASCT and nine patients with MM not suitable for HDT.[64] A significant

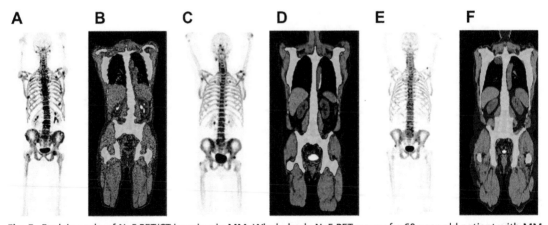

Fig. 5. Evolving role of NaF PET/CT imaging in MM. Whole-body NaF PET scans of a 60-year-old patient with MM that demonstrates multiple focal abnormalities throughout the skeleton (*A*). CT-based segmentation of bony skeleton allows global measurement of Na uptake for assessing osseous structures (*B*). In this patient with smoldering MM, NaF PET scan revealed minimal skeletal lesions (*C*). CT-based segmentation allows quantification of NaF uptake in various skeletal structures (*C, D*). NaF PET image of a healthy control subject and the corresponding segmented PET/CT scans (*E, F*) (OsiriX software, Pixmeo SARL, Bernex, Switzerland). The values are demonstrated in the table below.

GSUVmean	MM	SMM	Healthy Subject
	3.1	2.64	2.58

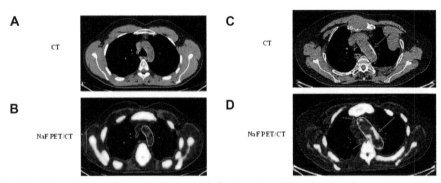

Fig. 6. NaF PET imaging to detect molecular calcification in atherosclerotic plaques. Normal NaF PET/CT in the thoracic aorta of a healthy subject (A, B) and The arrows show diffuse NaF uptake in the thoracic aorta of a patient with MM (C, D).

decrease in GSUVmean was observed after treatment with HDT, but no significant difference was observed after treatment in non-HDT patients, demonstrating that this technique is sensitive to show differences in the evaluation of response to therapy (**Fig. 4**).[64]

Moreover, this method of quantification was also used to analyze NaF PET/CT images in 35 patients with MM and nine patients with SMM in a prospective study and compared the results with 19 matched control subjects.[65] The global SUVmean, as measured by CT segmentation of the entire skeleton based on a fused PET/CT image, was significantly higher in MM than in SMM and healthy subjects (**Fig. 5**).[65] Thus, analysis of NaF PET was able to show difference in bone remodeling among MM, SMM, and healthy subjects. The higher NaF uptake in patients with MM indicates that bone destruction in patients with MM is followed by increased bone remodeling, which results in increased NaF uptake on PET.

THE ROLE OF SODIUM FLUORIDE IN ASSESSING ATHEROSCLEROSIS IN PATIENTS WITH MULTIPLE MYELOMA

Increasingly, high incidence of atherosclerosis is noted in patients diagnosed with several malignances as determined by conventional techniques.[66] Molecular imaging with PET is playing a major role in detecting and characterizing atherosclerotic plaques.[67] Calcification is one of the main features of atherosclerosis, and macroscopic calcification in the coronary and other arteries are identified by CT. However, CT is

neither able to detect active, early stage calcification or reliably differentiate vulnerable plaques from other types of plaques.[68] Uptake of NaF as a PET tracer reflects calcium deposition in tissues and is capable of detecting atherosclerosis in its early stages. Therefore, NaF PET/CT has the potential for cardiovascular risk stratification. In a preliminary study of 44 untreated myeloma patients and 26 healthy control subjects, regions of interest were assigned on NaF PET/CT images in the ascending aorta, aortic arch, and descending aorta. There was a significant difference between the average SUVmean in myeloma and control groups (**Fig. 6**). These preliminary results showed that the uptake of NaF in the thoracic aorta of myeloma patients was higher than that of the control group, which implies potential for NaF PET/CT to evaluate molecular calcification in plaques in patients with hematologic malignancy including MM.

SUMMARY

FDG PET/CT allows metabolic assessment of disease activity, which may prove to be superior to morphologic data derived from CT in patients with MM. Therefore, PET/CT can detect skeletal lesions and EMD, which can help physicians predict clinical course and assess the efficacy of therapy in this common hematologic malignancy. In particular, changes in FDG avidity provide an earlier indication of response as compared with MR imaging, so such changes are able to predict outcomes better than other imaging modalities, specifically in those who are candidates for ASCT. Moreover, external and internal MRD are detected using

FDG-PET/CT combined with sensitive bone marrow evaluation tools. DTPI is another technique that can be used in assessing FDG PET/CT scans of the patients with MM and differentiate between potential complete responders and those with partial response. Despite these promising roles, the use of PET in the clinical practice of monitoring patients with MM has been hampered by the lack of standardized methodologies that allow accurate and reproducible results. Finally, NaF imaging to assess skeletal abnormalities and calcification in the arteries of patients with myeloma disease may further enhance the role of PET imaging in this aggressive cancer. In this review, we have discussed approaches that may overcome the existing deficiencies of the current techniques.

ACKNOWLEDGEMENTS

All the works that are related to collaboration between the University of Pennsylvania and the University of Southern Denmark and mentioned in this review article were funded by the Region of Southern Denmark, University of Southern Denmark, Odense University Hospital, Harboe Foundation, The A.P.Møller Foundation (Fonden til lægevidenskabens fremme,), Aase & Ejnar Danielsen Foundation, The Family Hede Nielsen Foundation. The protocol was approved by the Danish Ethics Committee (S-20120209), the Danish Data Protection Agency (2008-58-0035) and registered at clinicaltrials.gov (NCT02187731). All patients gave written informed consent.

REFERENCES

1. Siegel RL, Miller KD, Jemal A. Cancer statistics, 2017. CA Cancer J Clin 2017;67(1):7–30.
2. Kumar SK, Rajkumar V, Kyle RA, et al. Multiple myeloma. Nat Rev Dis Primers 2017;3:17046.
3. Rajkumar SV, Dimopoulos MA, Palumbo A, et al. International Myeloma Working Group updated criteria for the diagnosis of multiple myeloma. Lancet Oncol 2014;15(12):e538–48.
4. Sonneveld P, Broijl A. Treatment of relapsed and refractory multiple myeloma. Haematologica 2016; 101(4):396–406.
5. Terpos E, Dimopoulos M-A. Myeloma bone disease: pathophysiology and management. Ann Oncol 2005;16(8):1223–31.
6. Valentin-Opran A, Charhon SA, Meunier PJ, et al. Quantitative histology of myeloma-induced bone changes. Br J Haematol 1982;52(4):601–10.
7. Taube T, Beneton MN, McCloskey EV, et al. Abnormal bone remodelling in patients with myelomatosis and normal biochemical indices of bone resorption. Eur J Haematol 1992;49(4):192–8.
8. Bataille R, Chappard D, Marcelli C, et al. Recruitment of new osteoblasts and osteoclasts is the earliest critical event in the pathogenesis of human multiple myeloma. J Clin Invest 1991;88(1):62–6.
9. Dimopoulos M, Terpos E, Comenzo RL, et al. International myeloma working group consensus statement and guidelines regarding the current role of imaging techniques in the diagnosis and monitoring of multiple myeloma. Leukemia 2009;23(9):1545–56.
10. D'Sa S, Abildgaard N, Tighe J, et al. Guidelines for the use of imaging in the management of myeloma. Br J Haematol 2007;137(1):49–63.
11. Edelstyn GA, Gillespie PJ, Grebbell FS. The radiological demonstration of osseous metastases. Experimental observations. Clin Radiol 1967;18(2): 158–62.
12. Cavo M, Terpos E, Nanni C, et al. Role of (18)F-FDG PET/CT in the diagnosis and management of multiple myeloma and other plasma cell disorders: a consensus statement by the International Myeloma Working Group. Lancet Oncol 2017; 18(4):e206–17.
13. Raynor W, Houshmand S, Gholami S, et al. Evolving role of molecular imaging with (18)F-sodium fluoride PET as a biomarker for calcium metabolism. Curr Osteoporos Rep 2016;14(4):115–25.
14. Ayubcha C, Zirakchian Zadeh M, Stochkendahl MJ, et al. Quantitative evaluation of normal spinal osseous metabolism with 18F-NaF PET/CT. Nucl Med Commun 2018;39(10):945–50.
15. Segall G, Delbeke D, Stabin MG, et al. SNM practice guideline for sodium 18F-fluoride PET/CT bone scans 1.0. J Nucl Med 2010;51(11):1813–20.
16. Beheshti M, Mottaghy FM, Paycha F, et al. (18)F-NaF PET/CT: EANM procedure guidelines for bone imaging. Eur J Nucl Med Mol Imaging 2015;42(11): 1767–77.
17. Grant FD, Fahey FH, Packard AB, et al. Skeletal PET with 18F-fluoride: applying new technology to an old tracer. J Nucl Med 2008;49(1):68–78.
18. Wahl RL, Jacene H, Kasamon Y, et al. From RECIST to PERCIST: evolving considerations for PET response criteria in solid tumors. J Nucl Med 2009; 50(Suppl 1):122S.
19. Boellaard R. The engagement of FDG PET/CT image quality and harmonized quantification: from competitive to complementary. Eur J Nucl Med Mol Imaging 2016;43(1):1–4.
20. Ziai P, Hayeri MR, Salei A, et al. Role of optimal quantification of FDG PET imaging in the clinical practice of radiology. Radiographics 2016;36(2): 481–96.
21. Zaidi H, Alavi A. Trends in PET quantification: opportunities and challenges. Clin Transl Imaging 2014; 2(3):183–5.
22. Baur-Melnyk A, Buhmann S, Becker C, et al. Whole-body MRI versus whole-body MDCT for staging of

multiple myeloma. AJR Am J Roentgenol 2008; 190(4):1097–104.

23. Lutje S, de Rooy JW, Croockewit S, et al. Role of radiography, MRI and FDG-PET/CT in diagnosing, staging and therapeutical evaluation of patients with multiple myeloma. Ann Hematol 2009;88(12): 1161–8.

24. Van Lammeren-Venema D1, Regelink JC, Riphagen II, et al. ^{18}F-fluoro-deoxyglucose positron emission tomography in assessment of myeloma-related bone disease: a systematic review. Cancer 2012;118(8):1971–81.

25. Zamagni E, Nanni C, Patriarca F, et al. A prospective comparison of 18F-fluorodeoxyglucose positron emission tomography-computed tomography, magnetic resonance imaging and whole-body planar radiographs in the assessment of bone disease in newly diagnosed multiple myeloma. Haematologica 2007;92(1):50–5.

26. Fonti R, Salvatore B, Quarantelli M, et al. 18F-FDG PET/CT, 99mTc-MIBI, and MRI in evaluation of patients with multiple myeloma. J Nucl Med 2008; 49(2):195.

27. Sachpekidis C, Mai EK, Goldschmidt H, et al. 18F-FDG dynamic PET/CT in patients with multiple myeloma: patterns of tracer uptake and correlation with bone marrow plasma cell infiltration rate. Clin Nucl Med 2015;40(6):e300–7.

28. Nanni C, Zamagni E, Farsad M, et al. Role of 18 F-FDG PET/CT in the assessment of bone involvement in newly diagnosed multiple myeloma: preliminary results. Eur J Nucl Med Mol Imaging 2006; 33(5):525–31.

29. Breyer RJ, Mulligan ME, Smith SE, et al. Comparison of imaging with FDG PET/CT with other imaging modalities in myeloma. Skeletal Radiol 2006;35(9):632–40.

30. Hur J, Yoon CS, Ryu YH, et al. Comparative study of fluorodeoxyglucose positron emission tomography and magnetic resonance imaging for the detection of spinal bone marrow infiltration in untreated patients with multiple myeloma. Acta Radiol 2008; 49(4):427–35.

31. Sager S, Ergül N, Ciftci H, et al. The value of FDG PET/CT in the initial staging and bone marrow involvement of patients with multiple myeloma. Skeletal Radiol 2011;40(7):843–7.

32. Spinnato P, Bazzocchi A, Brioli A, et al. Contrast enhanced MRI and 18F-FDG PET-CT in the assessment of multiple myeloma: a comparison of results in different phases of the disease. Eur J Radiol 2012; 81(12):4013–8.

33. Bredella MA, Steinbach L, Caputo G, et al. Value of FDG PET in the assessment of patients with multiple myeloma. Am J Roentgenol 2005;184(4):1199–204.

34. Regelink JC, Minnema MC, Terpos E, et al. Comparison of modern and conventional imaging techniques in establishing multiple myeloma-related

bone disease: a systematic review. Br J Haematol 2013;162(1):50–61.

35. Moreau P, Attal M, Caillot D, et al. Prospective evaluation of MRI and PET-CT at diagnosis and before maintenance therapy in symptomatic patients with multiple myeloma included in the IFM/DFCI 2009 trial. J Clin Oncol 2015;35(25):2911–8.

36. Sachpekidis C, Goldschmidt H, Hose D, et al. PET/CT studies of multiple myeloma using (18) F-FDG and (18) F-NaF: comparison of distribution patterns and tracers' pharmacokinetics. Eur J Nucl Med Mol Imaging 2014;41(7):1343–53.

37. Ak I, Onner H, Akay OM. Is there any complimentary role of F-18 NaF PET/CT in detecting of osseous involvement of multiple myeloma? A comparative study for F-18 FDG PET/CT and F-18 FDG NaF PET/CT. Ann Hematol 2015;94(9):1567–75.

38. Oral A, Yazici B, Ömür Ö, et al. 18F-FDG and 18F-NaF PET/CT findings of a multiple myeloma patient with thyroid cartilage involvement. Clin Nucl Med 2015;40(11):873–6.

39. Ak I, Gulbas Z. F-18 FDG uptake of bone marrow on PET/CT scan: it's correlation with CD38/CD138 expressing myeloma cells in bone marrow of patients with multiple myeloma. Ann Hematol 2011;90(1): 81–7.

40. Hillner BE, Siegel BA, Shields AF, et al. Relationship between cancer type and impact of PET and PET/CT on intended management: findings of the national oncologic PET registry. J Nucl Med 2008;49(12): 1928.

41. Zamagni E, Patriarca F, Nanni C, et al. Prognostic relevance of 18-F FDG PET/CT in newly diagnosed multiple myeloma patients treated with up-front autologous transplantation. Blood 2011;118(23): 5989–95.

42. Bartel TB, Haessler J, Brown TL, et al. F18-fluorodeoxyglucose positron emission tomography in the context of other imaging techniques and prognostic factors in multiple myeloma. Blood 2009;114(10): 2068–76.

43. Fonti R, Larobina M, Del Vecchio S, et al. Metabolic tumor volume assessed by 18F-FDG PET/CT for the prediction of outcome in patients with multiple myeloma. J Nucl Med 2012;53(12):1829.

44. Haznedar R, Akı SZ, Akdemir OU, et al. Value of 18 F-fluorodeoxyglucose uptake in positron emission tomography/computed tomography in predicting survival in multiple myeloma. Eur J Nucl Med Mol Imaging 2011;38(6):1046–53.

45. Zamagni E, Nanni C, Mancuso K, et al. PET/CT improves the definition of complete response and allows to detect otherwise unidentifiable skeletal progression in multiple myeloma. Clin Cancer Res 2015;21(19):4384–90.

46. Patriarca F, Carobolante F, Zamagni E, et al. The role of positron emission tomography with 18F-

fluorodeoxyglucose integrated with computed to-mography in the evaluation of patients with multiple myeloma undergoing allogeneic stem cell transplantation. Biol Blood Marrow Transplant 2015;21(6):1068–73.

47. Lapa C, Lückerath K, Malzahn U, et al. 18FDG-PET/CT for prognostic stratification of patients with multiple myeloma relapse after stem cell transplantation. Oncotarget 2014;5(17):7381.

48. Usmani SZ, Mitchell A, Waheed S, et al. Prognostic implications of serial 18-fluoro-deoxyglucose emission tomography in multiple myeloma treated with total therapy 3. Blood 2013;121(10):1819–23.

49. Dimitrakopoulou-Strauss A, Hoffmann M, Bergner R, et al. Prediction of progression-free survival in patients with multiple myeloma following anthracycline-based chemotherapy based on dynamic FDG-PET. Clin Nucl Med 2009;34(9):576–84.

50. Beksac M, Gunduz M, Ozen M, et al. Impact of PET-CT response on survival parameters following autologous stem cell transplantation among patients with multiple myeloma: comparison of two cut-off values. Blood 2014;124(21):3983.

51. Korde N, Roschewski M, Zingone A, et al. Treatment with carfilzomib-lenalidomide-dexamethasone with lenalidomide extension in patients with smoldering or newly diagnosed multiple myeloma. JAMA Oncol 2015;1(6):746–54.

52. Nanni C, Zamagni E, Celli M, et al. The value of 18F-FDG PET/CT after autologous stem cell transplantation (ASCT) in patients affected by multiple myeloma (MM): experience with 77 patients. Clin Nucl Med 2013;38(2):e74–9.

53. Cascini GL, Falcone C, Console D, et al. Whole-body MRI and PET/CT in multiple myeloma patients during staging and after treatment: personal experience in a longitudinal study. Radiol Med 2013;118(6):930–48.

54. Kumar S, Paiva B, Anderson KC, et al. International Myeloma Working Group consensus criteria for response and minimal residual disease assessment in multiple myeloma. Lancet Oncol 2016;17(8):e328–46.

55. Munshi NC, Avet-Loiseau H, Rawstron AC, et al. Association of minimal residual disease with superior survival outcomes in patients with multiple myeloma: a meta-analysis. JAMA Oncol 2017;3(1):28–35.

56. Raynor WY, Al-Zaghal A, Zadeh MZ, et al. Metastatic seeding attacks bone marrow, not bone: rectifying ongoing misconceptions. PET Clin 2019;14(1):135–44.

57. Basu S, Kung J, Houseni M, et al. Temporal profile of fluorodeoxyglucose uptake in malignant lesions and normal organs over extended time periods in patients with lung carcinoma: implications for its utilization in assessing malignant lesions. Q J Nucl Med Mol Imaging 2009;53(1):9.

58. Boerner A, Weckesser M, Herzog H, et al. Optimal scan time for fluorine-18 fluorodeoxyglucose positron emission tomography in breast cancer. Eur J Nucl Med 1999;26(3):226–30.

59. Houshmand S, Salavati A, Segtnan EA, et al. Dual-time-point imaging and delayed-time-point fluorodeoxyglucose-PET/computed tomography imaging in various clinical settings. PET Clin 2016;11(1):65–84.

60. Kumar R, Loving VA, Chauhan A, et al. Potential of dual-time-point imaging to improve breast cancer diagnosis with 18F-FDG PET. J Nucl Med 2005;46(11):1819–24.

61. Taghvaei R, Oestergaard B, Zadeh MZ, et al. Correlation of dual time point FDG-PET with response to chemotherapy in multiple myeloma. J Nucl Med 2017;58(supplement 1):188.

62. Alavi A, Werner TJ, Høilund-Carlsen PF, et al. Correction for partial volume effect is a must, not a luxury, to fully exploit the potential of quantitative PET imaging in clinical oncology. Mol Imaging Biol 2018;20(1):1–3.

63. Raynor W, Zadeh MZ, Acosta-Montenegro O, et al. Measuring bone marrow activity with FDG-PET in multiple myeloma, smoldering myeloma, and healthy subjects. J Nucl Med 2018;59(supplement 1):1420.

64. Zadeh MZ, Raynor W, Oestergaard B, et al. Changes in bone marrow FDG uptake in multiple myeloma patients before and after treatment. J Nucl Med 2018;59(supplement 1):1430.

65. Raynor W, Zadeh MZ, Acosta-Montenegro O, et al. Systemic bone remodeling in multiple myeloma, smoldering myeloma, and healthy subjects: global assessment with NaF-PET. J Nucl Med 2018;59(supplement 1):24.

66. Koene RJ, Prizment AE, Blaes A, et al. Shared risk factors in cardiovascular disease and cancer. Circulation 2016;133(11):1104–14.

67. Rosa GM, Bauckneht M, Masoero G, et al. The vulnerable coronary plaque: update on imaging technologies. Thromb Haemost 2013;110(4):706–22.

68. Huang H, Virmani R, Younis H, et al. The impact of calcification on the biomechanical stability of atherosclerotic plaques. Circulation 2001;103(8):1051–6.

Response-Adapted Treatment Strategies in Hodgkin Lymphoma Using PET Imaging

Steven M. Bair, MD*, Jakub Svoboda, MD

KEYWORDS

- Hodgkin lymphoma • Response-adapted • PET • Prognostic

KEY POINTS

- In Hodgkin lymphoma, there is a need to minimize the long-term toxicities of standard therapy without sacrificing the gains that have been made in efficacy.
- An expanding body of literature supports a role for FDG-PET in guiding therapy for certain patients with Hodgkin lymphoma.
- Technical limitations inherent to FDG-PET introduce challenges into response-adapted treatment strategies.

INTRODUCTION

Approximately 8500 new cases of Hodgkin lymphoma (HL) are diagnosed in the United States every year, comprising about 10% of all new lymphoma diagnoses.[1] In the developed world, new cases of HL occur along a bimodal age distribution with a large peak in incidence around age 20 and a smaller peak after age 65. Seventy percent of new cases occur in individuals less than 55 years of age.[2]

HL is derived from germinal center or postgerminal center B cells and is characterized by unique clinicopathologic features. The tumor microenvironment plays a critical role in the development and progression of HL, as well as the response to treatment.[3,4] For example, the malignant cells in HL, Reed-Sternberg cells, comprise less than 1% of the tumor volume, but they are immersed in a complex inflammatory milieu that drives immune dysregulation, tumor cell evasion of the immune system, and disease progression.[5–9]

Over the last several decades, HL has been transformed from a universally fatal malignancy[10,11] to a highly curable disease with current frontline and salvage treatment approaches. Doxorubicin, bleomycin, vinblastine, and dacarbazine (ABVD) with or without radiotherapy is the most common frontline treatment regimen, resulting in overall long-term complete remission rates of almost 80%.[12,13] Escalated-dose bleomycin, etoposide, doxorubicin, cyclophosphamide, vincristine, procarbazine, and prednisone (eBEACOPP) is another highly effective regimen with more potent antilymphoma activity, but greater toxicity, that is primarily used outside the United

Disclosures: No disclosures (S.M. Bair). Merck: Research Funding; Regeneron: Research Funding; Kyowa: Consultancy; TG Therapeutics: Research Funding; Pharmacyclics: Consultancy, Research Funding; Bristol-Myers Squibb: Consultancy, Research Funding; KITE: Consultancy; Seattle Genetics: Consultancy, Research Funding (J. Svoboda).
Lymphoma Program, Abramson Cancer Center, University of Pennsylvania, 3400 Civic Center Boulevard, PCAM 12th Floor, South Extension, Philadelphia, PA 19104, USA
* Corresponding author.
E-mail address: steven.bair@uphs.upenn.edu

PET Clin 14 (2019) 353–368
https://doi.org/10.1016/j.cpet.2019.03.008
1556-8598/19/© 2019 Elsevier Inc. All rights reserved.

States. Patients with early-stage disease (stage I/II) achieve 5-year progression-free survival (PFS) rates of greater than 90%.[14] Patients with advanced disease (stage III/IV) experience slightly worse outcomes with 5-year PFS ranging between 70% and 90% depending on the population and treatment regimen studied.[13,15,16]

Although the standard management of HL produces cures in most patients, these chemotherapy and radiotherapy regimens are not without significant short- and long-term toxicities. Patients with HL are more likely to die from toxicity of antilymphoma treatment or other unrelated causes than from HL.[17,18] Following treatment of HL (especially combined modality therapy), survivors are more likely than the general population to experience secondary malignancies, such as breast cancer,[19–23] gastrointestinal cancer,[24,25] and lung cancer.[26–28] More aggressive regimens, are associated with a higher risk of developing treatment-related myelodysplasia or acute myeloid leukemia, which carries a dismal prognosis.[29,30] In addition to secondary malignancies, these patients have a higher risk of coronary artery disease, which is associated with the dose of mediastinal radiation,[31] a higher incidence of long-term pulmonary dysfunction,[32] and increased rates of infertility.[33,34]

The challenge of treating patients with HL in the modern era, therefore, is to maximize the benefits of the highly effective regimens that have evolved over the last 50 years, while minimizing the short-term and long-term toxicities. This imperative has led to a strong interest in predicting, early in the course of therapy, those patients who might benefit from de-escalation of therapy without loss of disease control and, conversely, predicting those patients in whom intensification of therapy would provide a benefit. This review summarizes the various "response-adapted" treatment approaches that have been studied in both early-stage and advanced-stage HL. We also discuss PET imaging, the most commonly used modality in response-adapted protocols.

^{18}F-FLUORO-2-DEOXY-D-GLUCOSE-PET IN HODGKIN LYMPHOMA

Upregulation of glycolytic pathways in proliferating tumor cells results in an increase in glucose transport proteins on the cell surface and increased expression of intracellular glycolytic enzymes, thereby allowing increased flux through glycolytic pathways. ^{18}F-Fluoro-2-deoxy-D-glucose (FDG) is a synthetic glucose analog that is administered via intravenous injection and is taken up into metabolically active cells, where it becomes phosphorylated and is retained in the cytoplasm. FDG can be detected and quantified using PET. This modality has become widely used in oncology to stage and assess treatment response in a variety of tumors.

The first studies describing the use of FDG-PET in lymphoma were published in the 1990s.[35,36] In the 2000s, accumulating evidence suggested that FDG-PET could be used to monitor treatment response and that, when performed early in the course of treatment (termed interim-PET), it had prognostic significance. A 2005 retrospective analysis of patients with HL who had undergone interim-PET imaging after 2 to 3 cycles of therapy demonstrated that FDG-PET could be used not only to detect early response to therapy but also to predict outcomes.[37] Several subsequent studies prospectively demonstrated the ability of FDG-PET to predict treatment response and long-term outcomes.[38–40] For example, Gallamini and colleagues[39] published a study of interim-PET after 2 cycles (PET2) of ABVD in 205 patients primarily with advanced HL and reported 2-year PFS rates of 95% and 13% among patients with PET2-negative and PET2-positive disease, respectively. In this study, the status of the interim-PET scan was more predictive of 2-year PFS than the International Prognostic Score and the presence of extranodal or bulky disease. These early studies laid the foundation for subsequent work evaluating response-adapted treatment approaches.

As FDG-PET came into more widespread use for the diagnosis and management of lymphomas, a standardized approach to interpretation was needed. In 2007, the International Harmonization Project (IHP) criteria were developed to standardize the interpretation of FDG-PET.[41] These criteria defined residual disease as a residual mass greater than 2 cm with FDG uptake intensity greater than that of the mediastinal blood pool and for masses ≤2 cm, FDG uptake intensity greater than background. In 2009, the First International Workshop on PET in Lymphoma met in Deauville, France, and proposed a new 5-point scoring system that came to be known as the Deauville criteria (**Table 1**).[42] Scores of 4 or 5 represent uptake moderately or markedly higher than the liver, respectively, or the presence of a new lesion (Deauville 5), and is considered positive. In 2014, the Deauville criteria were formally incorporated into the Lugano classification system for malignant lymphoma.[43] More recently, the international Response Evaluation Criteria in Lymphoma (RECIL 2017) have proposed an assessment system that aligns more closely with the RECIST (Response Evaluation Criteria in Solid Tumors) system, is

Table 1
Deauville response criteria

Score	Description
1	No uptake
2	Uptake ≤ mediastinum
3	Uptake > mediastinum, but ≤ liver
4	Uptake moderately higher than liver
5	Uptake markedly higher than liver and/or new lesions

applicable to both adult and pediatric patients, and redefines response criteria, including the introduction of a "minor response category."[44] The RECIL 2017 criteria will require further validation in prospective studies. Whereas most studies of response-adapted therapy have used the Deauville criteria to determine interim-PET positivity, several studies have used other criteria. Even among studies that have applied the Deauville criteria, variation exists in how PET positivity is defined. **Tables 2** and **3** provide summaries of the clinical trials of response-adapted therapy in early-stage and advanced-stage HL, respectively, including the definition of PET positivity used in each trial.

RESPONSE-ADAPTED THERAPY IN EARLY-STAGE HODGKIN LYMPHOMA

Early-stage HL carries an excellent prognosis and a cure rate greater than 90% with standard initial therapy.[14] Even among patients who relapse, many can be effectively treated with salvage therapy with no decrement in rates of overall survival (OS). Therefore, most studies of response-adapted therapy in early HL (see **Table 2**) have focused on reducing the number of cycles of chemotherapy during initial treatment or eliminating radiotherapy in patients with a negative interim-PET. Only 1 randomized trial has evaluated treatment intensification in patients with early-stage, unfavorable HL in the context of a positive interim-PET.

The EORTC/LYSA/FIL H10F/U trial was one of the first randomized phase 3 trials of response-adapted therapy in early HL. The primary aim of this study was to assess whether involved node radiation therapy (INRT) could be safely omitted in patients with a negative interim-PET after 2 cycles of ABVD.[45] The study was designed as a noninferiority trial and a total of 1137 patients were included in the interim analysis, of which 444 had favorable-risk disease. Eighty-six percent (381 patients) had a negative

interim-PET2 and were randomized to receive either 1 additional cycle of ABVD followed by 30 Gy INRT (standard arm) or 2 additional cycles of ABVD (experimental arm). A preplanned interim analysis by the independent data monitoring committee recommended termination of the study due to futility because this analysis revealed a significant difference in disease progression between the 2 arms (1 in standard arm, 9 in experimental arm; hazard ratio [HR] = 9.36, 80% CI: 2.4–35.7). One-year PFS was 100% and 94.9% in the standard and experimental arms, respectively. Following the interim analysis, the experimental ABVD-only arm was closed. The final results of the H10 study were subsequently published,[46] demonstrating that among patients with favorable disease and a negative interim-PET2, there is superior rate of PFS in the standard combined modality therapy arm (5-year PFS 99% vs 87%; HR = 15.8, 95% CI: 3.8–66.1). These results support a continued role for consolidative radiation therapy (RT) in maintaining disease control in early-stage HL. Differences in OS were not observed.

The British RAPID trial[17] primarily enrolled patients with favorable-risk (stage IA/IIA) disease and sought to determine whether RT could be safely omitted following a negative interim-PET after 3 cycles of ABVD. The study enrolled 602 patients, of whom 75% had negative interim-PET3 and were randomly assigned to receive either INRT or no further therapy. Rates of 3-year PFS in the intention-to-treat analysis were 95% and 91% in the INRT and no treatment arms, respectively, although this difference was slightly larger in the per protocol analysis (6.3%). The study endpoints did not meet the prespecified margin for noninferiority, supporting a continued role for consolidative RT in most patients with early favorable disease.

Final results of the German Hodgkin Study Group (GSHG) HD16 trial were recently presented[47] and were consistent with the results of H10 and RAPID. Specifically, the goal of this study was also to determine whether radiotherapy could be safely omitted in patients with early favorable HL. These investigators reported that, among patients with a negative interim-PET who received 2 cycles of ABVD followed by 20 Gy involved field radiation therapy (IFRT), the 5-year PFS was 93% compared with 86% in patients treated with 2 cycles of ABVD alone. The difference in 5-year PFS was 7.3% (HR = 1.78; 95% CI: 1.03–3.21). There was a significant difference in the rate of in-field recurrence among patients in the combined modality and ABVD alone arms (2.1% vs 8.7%, respectively).

Table 2
Studies of PET-adapted therapy in early-stage Hodgkin lymphoma

Source	Trial	Clinical Stage	Initial Therapy	Definition of PET Positivity	Interim-PET Result	#/Arm	Risk-Adapted Treatment	Progression-Free Survival	Overall Survival
Radford et al,[17] 2015	RAPID	Early, favorable (stage IA/IIA)	3× ABVD followed by PET	DS 3–5	PET3–: 426/571 (75%)	211	No further therapy	3 y: 91% (87%–95%)	3 y: 99% (98%–100%)
						209	30 Gy IFRT	3 y: 95% (92%–98%)	3 y: 97% (95%–99%)
					PET3+: 145/571 (25%)	145	1× ABVD + IFRT	NR	NR
André et al,[46] 2017	EORTC/LYSA/FIL H10	Early-stage (I/II), favorable	2× ABVD followed by PET	IHP criteria	Favorable. PET2–: 465/562 (83%)	227	1 cycle ABVD + INRT	5 y: 99% (96%–100%)	5 y: 100% (na)
						238	2 cycles ABVD	5 y: 87% (82%–91%)	5 y: 99% (97%–100%)
		Early-stage (I/II), unfavorable			Unfavorable. PET2–: 594/858 (70%)	292	2× ABVD + INRT	5 y: 92% (88%–95%)	5 y: 97% (94%–98%)
						302	4× ABVD	5y: 90% (85%–93%)	5y: 98% (96%–99%)
André et al,[46] 2017	EORTC/LYSA/FIL H10	Early-stage (I/II), both favorable and unfavorable	2× ABVD followed by PET	IHP criteria	PET2+: 361/1925 (19%)	192	2× ABVD + INRT	5 y: 77% (70%–83%)	5 y: 89% (83%–93%)
						169	2× eBEACOPP + INRT	5 y: 91% (85%–94%)	5 y: 96% (91%–98%)
Straus et al,[48] 2018	CALGB 50604	Early-stage (I/II), both favorable and unfavorable, nonbulky	2× ABVD followed by PET	DS 4–5	PET2–: 135/149 (91%)	135	2× ABVD (no INRT)	3 y: 91%	NR
					PET2+: 14/149 (9%)	14	2× eBEACOPP + 3060 cGy IFRT	3 y: 66%	NR
Fuchs et al,[47] 2018	HD16	Early-stage (I/II), favorable	2× ABVD followed by PET	DS 3–5	Only PET2 patients randomized	328	20 Gy IFRT	5 y: 93% (90%–96%)	5 y: 98%
						300	No IFRT	5 y: 86% (81%–91%)	5 y: 98%

Abbreviations: DS, Deauville score; IFRT, involved field radiation therapy; INRT, involved node radiation therapy; NR, not reported.

Table 3
Studies of PET-adapted therapy in advanced-stage Hodgkin lymphoma

Source	Trial	Clinical Stage	Initial Therapy	Definition of PET Positivity	Interim-PET Result	N/Arm	Risk-Adapted Treatment	Progression-Free Survival/ Event-Free Survival	Overall Survival
Ganesan et al,[56] 2015	NCT01348490	High-risk stage IIB, III, or IV	2× ABVD followed by PET	DS 4–5	PET2–: 42/50 (84%)	42	4× ABVD	2 y EFS: 82%	NR
					PET2+: 8/50 (16%)	8	4× eBEACOPP	2 y EFS: 50%	NR
Johnson et al,[18] 2016	RATHL	Early or advanced; newly diagnosed patients	2× ABVD followed by PET	DS 4–5	PET2–: 937/1135 (83%)	470	4× ABVD	3 y: 86% (82%–89%)	3 y: 97% (95%–98%)
						465	4× ABVD with omission of bleomycin (AVD) in cycles 3–6	3 y: 84% (81%–87%)	3 y: 98% (96%–99%)
					PET2+: 182/1135 (16%)	172	BEACOPP14 or eBEACOPP	3 y: 67% (60%–74%)	3 y: 87% (81%–92%)
Press et al,[55] 2016	SWOG 0816	Stage III or IV	2× ABVD followed by PET	DS 4–5	PET2–: 271/331 (82%)	271	4× ABVD	2 y: 82% (77%–86%)	NR
					PET2+: 60/331 (18%)	60	6× eBEACOPP	2 y: 64% (50%–75%)	NR
Zinzani et al,[57] 2016	FIL HD0801	High-risk stage IIB, III, or IV	2× ABVD followed by PET	IHP	PET2–: 409/512 (80%)	409	4× ABVD	2 y: 81% (76%–84%)	NR
					PET2+: 103/512 (20%)	103	Ifosfamide-based salvage chemotherapy (eg, IGEV) followed by BEAM-conditioned ASCT	2 y: 76% (66–84)	NR

(continued on next page)

Table 3
(continued)

Source	Trial	Clinical Stage	Initial Therapy	Definition of PET Positivity	Interim-PET Result	N/Arm	Risk-Adapted Treatment	Progression-Free Survival/ Event-Free Survival	Overall Survival
Borchmann et al,[59] 2017	HD18	High-risk stage IIB, III, or IV	2× eBEACOPP followed by PET	DS 3–5	PET2–: 1013/1964 (51%)	504	4× or 6× eBEACOPP	5 y: 91% (90%–94%)	5 y: 95% (93%–97%)
						501	2× eBEACOPP	5 y: 92% (89%–95%)	5 y: 98% (96%–99%)
					PET2+: 951/1964 (48%)	217	6× eBEACOPP	5y: 90% (85%–94%)	5y: 97% (95%–99%)
						217	6× eBEACOPP + rituximab	5 y: 88% (83%–94%)	5 y: 94% (91%–97%)
Casasnovas et al,[58] 2018	LYSA AHL2011	High-risk stage IIB, III, or IV	6× eBEACOPP 2× eBEACOPP followed by PET	DS 4–5	N/A; standard treatment arm	413	N/A; standard treatment arm	5 y: 86.2%	NR
					PET2–: 346/410 (87%)	346	4× ABVD	Combined 5 y: 85.7%	NR
					PET2+: 51/410 (13%)	51	4× eBEACOPP	PET2– 5y: 88.9% PET2+ 5 y: 70.7%	NR
Gallamini et al,[54] 2018	GITIL/FIL HD 0607	High-risk stage IIB, III, or IV	2× ABVD followed by PET	DS 4–5	PET2–: 631/782 (81%)	631	4× ABVD (+/– RT)	3 y: 87%	99% 3 y-OS
					PET2+: 150/782 (19%)	150	4× eBEACOPP + 4× BEACOPP (+/– rituximab)	3 y: 60%	89% 3 y-OS

Abbreviations: BEAM, carmustine, etoposide, cytarabine, melphalan; DS, Deauville score; IGEV, ifosfamide, gemcitabine, and vinorelbine; N/A, not applicable; NR, not reported.

Finally, the US Intergroup (CALGB/Alliance) 50604 trial[48] aimed to describe the rates of PFS and OS when RT is omitted in the setting of a negative interim-PET. Patients (N = 149) with stage I/II, favorable or unfavorable (but nonbulky) HL were enrolled and treated with 2 cycles of ABVD followed by an interim-PET. Those with a negative PET2 received 2 additional doses of ABVD (without RT) followed by observation. Those with PET-positive disease after 2 cycles were switched to eBEACOPP for 2 cycles followed by 30 Gy IFRT. The 3-year PFS rates for the PET2-negative and PET2-positive patients were 91% and 66%, respectively, and no difference in OS was observed. The results suggest that the omission of radiotherapy after 4 cycles of ABVD in patients with early-stage, nonbulky HL and a negative interim-PET2 is still associated with excellent PFS, exceeding 90% at 3 years. However, the results of this study should be interpreted with caution given the lack of a comparison arm and in light of the H10, RAPID, and recent HD16 trial results. It is difficult to draw conclusions regarding therapy intensification following a positive PET2 because of the small number of patients (N = 14) including in this study.

The difference in the rate of 3-year PFS in RAPID (3.8%) and 5-year PFS in H10, and HD16 (11.9% and 7.3%, respectively), all favor combined modality therapy. Taken together, these results demonstrate that, among patients with early-stage disease, omission of RT on the basis of a negative interim-PET is more likely to result in loss of disease control, and that combined modality approaches should remain the standard for most patients when the primary goal is long-term disease control. However, an individualized approach in certain situations may be reasonable (**Fig. 1**). Among the clinical trials that have investigated de-escalation of therapy in patients with early-stage HL, no differences in OS have been observed.

Only 1 randomized clinical trial has evaluated intensification of treatment in patients with early-stage HL with positive interim-PET. A secondary aim of the H10 trial (discussed above) was to evaluate a strategy of response-adapted treatment intensification. In the standard arm, patients with favorable or unfavorable disease and a positive PET2 were treated with 1 or 2 cycles, respectively, of ABVD followed by INRT. Patients in the experimental arm were given 2 cycles of eBEACOPP followed by INRT. These investigators observed a significant benefit in favor of treatment intensification, with a significantly higher rate of PFS in the eBEACOPP arm (91% vs 77%; HR = 0.42, 95% CI: 0.23–0.74), as well as a numerically higher

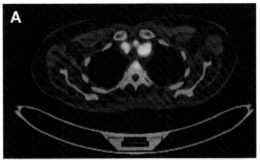

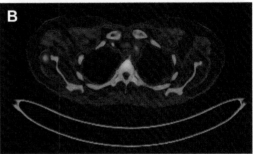

Fig. 1. A 45-year-old presented with left cervical lymphadenopathy and was diagnosed with stage IIA, favorable-risk classic HL. Pretreatment PET/CT demonstrated left cervical (A) and pericardiac lymphadenopathy. The patient was given ABVD and, after 2 cycles, an interim-PET/CT demonstrated complete metabolic response (B). The patient experienced nonspecific pulmonary symptoms. Given the negative interim-PET, bleomycin was omitted from cycles 3 and 4. Moreover, radiation therapy was believed to be high risk given the proximity to cardiac structures, so on the basis of the negative interim-PET and the potential for cardiac toxicity, radiation therapy was omitted. The patient remains in complete remission.

rate of OS (96% vs 89%), although this difference did not meet conventional thresholds for statistical significance. Interestingly, PET2-directed treatment intensification to 4 cycles eBEACOPP followed by INRT results in a rate of 5-year PFS similar to that observed in PET2-negative patients in the same study who continued with 4 additional cycles of ABVD followed by INRT (91% vs 92%, respectively). One limitation of this study was its use of IHP criteria in defining interim-PET positivity, which generally corresponds to a Deauville score (DS) of 3 to 5.[45] This may account, at least in part, for the high rates of PFS observed in this study because patients with DS 3 were more likely to be included in the intensification arm compared with other studies that used more stringent criteria to define PET positivity. Moreover, this approach likely increased the number of patients exposed to intensified treatment regimens unnecessarily.

Based on the above trial results, the National Comprehensive Cancer Network (NCCN)[49] and

European Society of Medical Oncology (ESMO)[50] guidelines recommend 2 cycles of ABVD followed by INRT for most patients with early-stage, favorable HL, although the NCCN guidelines also provide an alternative of 3 cycles of ABVD and omission of radiotherapy. For patients with early-stage, unfavorable HL, both sets of guidelines advocate for 4 cycles of ABVD or 2 cycles of ABVD intensified to eBEACOPP for 2 additional cycles, although consolidative radiotherapy should be included with either approach. Both sets of guidelines also provide the option of therapeutic intensification to eBEACOPP in the setting of a positive interim-PET.

RESPONSE-ADAPTED THERAPY IN ADVANCED HODGKIN LYMPHOMA

With standard frontline therapy, advanced HL can be cured in most cases. Previous studies have demonstrated rates of 5-year PFS of 68% to 85% depending on the regimen and population.[12,16,51–53] Escalated BEACOPP has been shown to produce higher rates of early disease control in advanced disease, but this PFS benefit has not translated to improved OS compared with ABVD and comes at the expense of greater treatment-related toxicity, both acute and chronic.[16] Studies of response-adapted therapy in advanced HL (see **Table 3**) have focused on both early intensification[18,54–57] and de-escalation[13,18,54,58,59] of therapy in patients with interim-PET-positive and PET-negative disease, respectively.

Therapy Intensification in Patients with Positive Interim-PET

The US Intergroup/Southwest Oncology Group S0816 study[55] was designed to test whether response-adapted therapy could improve on the rates of PFS observed with ABVD alone, and whether early intensification to BEACOPP in patients with positive interim-PET2 could improve outcomes in this high-risk population relative to historical controls.[39,60] Three hundred and fifty-eight patients with stage III-IV disease were enrolled and treated with 2 cycles of ABVD, followed by interim-PET. Patients with a positive PET2 (18%), were switched to eBEACOPP for 6 additional cycles. Those with a negative PET2 continued with an additional 4 cycles of ABVD. The rates of 2-year PFS among those with negative and positive PET2 were 82% and 64%, respectively. The latter demonstrated an improvement compared with historical controls. An extended follow-up analysis of S0816 was recently presented and reported 5-year PFS rates of 76%

and 65% in patients who were initially PET2-negative and PET2-positive, respectively.[61] The authors did find an increased rate of secondary malignancies in the patients who received eBEACOPP compared with ABVD (4% vs 2%; $P = .001$).

The Gruppo Italiano Terapie Innovative nei Linfomi (GITIL) HD0607 study evaluated the efficacy of early treatment intensification in patients with newly diagnosed advanced HL and a positive interim-PET.[54] Patients were treated with 2 cycles of ABVD, followed by PET2, which was centrally reviewed. Patients with positive PET2 went on to receive 4 cycles of eBEACOPP followed by 4 cycles of standard BEACOPP with or without rituximab. Patients with a negative PET2 completed a standard course of 6 cycles of ABVD. Five-year PFS and OS for the entire cohort was 82% and 97%, respectively, demonstrating that a response-adapted approach can result in rates of PFS and OS similar to those observed in previous studies of standard, nonresponse-adapted therapeutic approaches. There were lower rates of grades 3/4 hematologic toxicity (76% vs 30%) and infection (10% vs 1%) in patients who continued on ABVD compared with those who were escalated to BEACOPP. Patients with negative PET2 experienced improved rates of 5-year PFS and OS (87% and 99%, respectively) compared with patients who were PET2-positive (60% and 89%, respectively). The study also demonstrated that patients with a DS of 5 on PET2 had a markedly worse prognosis, with an estimated rate of 5-year PFS of only 35% (compared with 73% in those with DS of 4). Similar results were observed in the response-adapted therapy in Hodgkin lymphoma (RATHL) study (discussed below); 53% of patients with DS of 5 experienced disease progression within 3 years.[18] Together, the results of these studies suggest that patients with DS 5 on interim-PET are at high risk for relapse even in the setting of therapeutic intensification and innovative approaches are needed for this population.

The UK-led RATHL trial[18] was an international study to test whether interim-PET could be used to guide chemotherapy de-escalation (see later discussion) or intensification. Patients with newly diagnosed advanced HL were treated with 2 cycles of ABVD followed by interim-PET and those with a positive PET2 scan (17%) went on to receive either 3 or 4 cycles eBEACOPP or 4 to 6 cycles standard BEACOPP. Of the 1214 patients enrolled, 160 PET2-positive patients went on to receive eBEACOPP and 119 (74%) had a negative PET following treatment intensification. Patients who had a positive PET2 had 5-year PFS and OS rates of 67% and 88%, respectively, which are similar to rates observed in patients with positive interim-PET in other studies of PET-adapted therapy and higher than historical controls.[60,62]

Another approach to early response-adapted intensification was studied in the FIL HD0801 trial,[57] in which patients with advanced HL were treated with 2 cycles of ABVD, followed by interim-PET. Patients with a positive PET2 (20%) were treated with an ifosfamide-based salvage chemotherapy (ie, ifosfamide, gemcitabine, and vinorelbine), followed by carmustine, etoposide, cytarabine, melphalan-conditioned autologous stem cell transplant (ASCT). With this approach, the investigators reported a 2-year PFS of 76% in those with PET2-positive disease, which approaches the rate of PFS observed in PET2-negative patients in similar trials (see **Table 3**). Patients who were PET2-negative went on to receive an additional 4 cycles of ABVD. One limitation of this study, however, is that it was designed before the widespread adoption of the Deauville criteria and uses the IHP criteria for interim-PET assessment. Re-evaluation of the imaging studies using the Deauville criteria demonstrated that 30% of subjects had DS 3; the inclusion of a significant number of patients with DS 3 at interim-PET likely contributed to the increased survival. As that study only reported 2-year outcomes, more extended follow-up would provide additional insight regarding this therapeutic approach.

RATHL, S0816, and GITIL, all described above, show a consistent rate of 3-year PFS of approximately 60% to 67% in patients who are treated with intensified regimens because of a positive interim-PET. It should be noted that these studies evaluate the efficacy of eBEACOPP in the absence of a standard comparison arm because previous studies demonstrated that patients continued on ABVD after a positive interim-PET had 2-year PFS rates as low as 13%,[39,60] calling into question the clinical equipoise of including ABVD comparison arms in the design of these studies.

Taken together, these studies suggest that escalation of therapy in patients with a positive interim-PET is feasible and may produce superior rates of PFS when compared with historical controls. However, more intensive regimens such as BEACOPP or ASCT are associated with increased toxicity. Although these studies do provide evidence of improved disease control with response-adapted intensification of therapy, more data are needed to understand the long-term toxicities and complications as well as to understand whether OS differences will emerge with a response-adapted approach. In the absence of a clear standard, it is important to continue to

provide patients with opportunities to participate in clinical trials that address these questions. **Fig. 2** provides an example of therapeutic intensification in a patient with advanced classical Hodgkin lymphoma and persistent PET-positive disease.

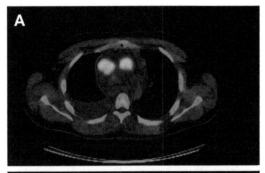

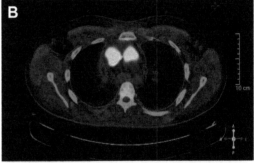

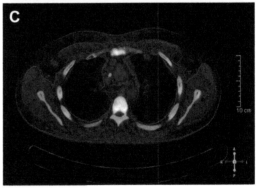

Fig. 2. A 22-year-old was diagnosed with stage IVB classic HL with several negative prognostic factors. The patient's initial PET/CT (*A*) was performed at a different center but is included here for comparison. The patient initially received 2 cycles of ABVD. PET/CT performed after 2 cycles was positive for persistent disease (*B*). Given the high-risk features and persistent PET-positive disease, therapy was changed to BEACOPP and, after 2 cycles of BEACOPP, repeat PET/CT demonstrated metabolic complete remission (CR) (*C*). The latter PET/CT demonstrated bone marrow uptake, but this was attributed to recent exposure to granulocyte colony-stimulating factor. The patient received a total of 4 cycles of BEACOPP followed by radiation therapy and remains in CR.

Therapy De-escalation in Patients with Negative Interim-PET

As discussed above, early retrospective studies evaluating the prognostic use of PET/computed tomography (CT) in advanced HL suggested that a negative interim-PET is strongly prognostic, and was associated with 3-year PFS rates as high as 95%.[39,60] Although more recent prospective studies have not demonstrated PFS rates as high as this, they consistently showed durable remission rates of 80% to 90%. Because of the relatively high negative predictive value of interim-PET in advanced HL, investigators became interested in therapy de-escalation in patients who were likely to respond to standard upfront therapy with the goal of reducing short-term and long-term toxicity. In general, studies looking at de-escalation have focused on (1) reducing the intensity of frontline therapy by switching from eBEACOPP to ABVD following a negative interim-PET, (2) reduction in the number of cycles of intensive therapy (ie, eBEACOPP), and (3) the safety of omitting consolidative RT.

The primary aim of RATHL was to evaluate whether interim-PET could be used to guide subsequent therapy. Patients enrolled in the RATHL study received 2 cycles of ABVD followed by an interim-PET, and those with a negative interim-PET (83%) continued ABVD for a total of 6 cycles but were randomized to receive either the full ABVD regimen or to omit bleomycin for cycles 3 to 6 (ie, AVD). There was no difference in the rate of relapse, progression, or death between the 2 arms (HR = 1.13; 95% CI: 0.81–1.57), and they demonstrated a nonsignificant −1.3% difference in 3-year PFS (85.7% vs 84.4% in ABVD vs AVD arms, respectively). Although the upper bound of the 95% CI of the difference was 5.3%, just exceeding the prespecified cutoff of 5.0%, the omission of bleomycin was associated with less of a decline in pulmonary function during therapy (7.4% reduction; 95% CI: 5.1–9.7; $P = .003$) that was sustained. In sum, the study demonstrated that, in patients with a negative interim-PET scan, omission of bleomycin is unlikely to increase the risk of progression, relapse, or death, but preserves pulmonary function. Based on these results, the NCCN[49] and ESMO[50] guidelines both recommend omission of bleomycin after 2 cycles of ABVD in the setting of a negative PET2.

The German Hodgkin Study Group (GHSG) designed the HD18 trial[59] to evaluate whether disease control could be maintained with fewer cycles of eBEACOPP. These investigators enrolled nearly 2000 patients, who were treated with 2 cycles of eBEACOPP, followed by an interim-PET.

Patients with a negative PET2 (51%) were randomized to receive either 4 to 6 additional cycles or only 2 further cycles of eBEACOPP. Patients with a positive PET2 went on to receive 4 to 6 cycles of eBEACOPP either alone or in combination with rituximab. All patients with nodal disease $\geq$2.5 cm also received RT. Of note, results of the HD15 study were reported while this trial was actively accruing, prompting a protocol amendment mandating a reduction in the total number of cycles of eBEACOPP from 8 to 6 cycles, therefore, patients randomized to the standard treatment arm after June 2011 received a maximum of 6 total cycles (rather than 8). A positive interim-PET in this study was defined as DS 3 to 5, rather than 4 to 5, as has been done in most other studies. In the negative PET2 arms, a similar rate of 5-year PFS was observed in those receiving a total of 4 compared 6 to 8 cycles of eBEACOPP (92% vs 91%, respectively). Rates of 5-year OS were also similar between the 2 groups (95% vs 98%). Patients who received fewer cycles of eBEACOPP, however, experienced a lower risk of severe infection (8% vs 15%) and organ toxicity (8% vs 18%). These investigators did not detect a difference in the risk of secondary malignancy between the 2 groups after a median of 5.5 years of follow-up. These results suggest that, in patients with advanced HL treated with eBEACOPP, 4 cycles result in similar disease control compared with either 6 or 8 cycles, but with a reduction in treatment-related toxicity.

The final results of the French LYSA AHL2011 study were recently reported[58] and is one of the few studies with a randomization arm to standard treatment without interim-PET. Four hundred and thirteen patients were randomized to receive 6 cycles of eBEACOPP without interim-PET, and the remaining 410 patients were randomized to initiate therapy with 2 cycles of eBEACOPP followed by interim-PET. Patients who were PET2-negative were switched to ABVD for an additional 4 cycles; patients who were PET2-positive continued with eBEACOPP for a total of 6 cycles. Rates of 5-year PFS did not differ between the standard and PET-adapted arms (both 86% vs 86%). Within the PET-adapted treatment arm, patients with a positive PET2 had significantly lower 5-year PFS compared with those who were PET2-negative (71% vs 89%, respectively). The authors reported a significantly lower rate of serious adverse events in patients treated with ABVD after 2 cycles of eBEACOPP compared with those who received 6 cycles of eBEACOPP (28% vs 45%). Both HD18 and LYSA2011 provide evidence that patients with advanced HL who are initiated on therapy with eBEACOPP can transition to a less intensive approach following negative interim-PET.

Although radiotherapy was initially the foundation of curative treatment approaches for HL, the increased efficacy of systemic therapies over the years and the recognition of the importance of reducing long-term toxicities, has led to a shift in the role of radiotherapy, especially in advanced HL. Radiotherapy has been associated with several late toxicities,[63–65] and recent studies evaluating the benefit of this modality in advanced HL have been conflicting.[66–70] The GHSG HD15 trial was designed to include RT only for those with a residual bulky mass and PET positivity after completion of frontline chemotherapy.[13] The authors noted 11% of patients in this study underwent a course of consolidative radiotherapy using this protocol, compared with 71% in the previous GHSG HD9 trial, while maintaining excellent rates of 5-year PFS and OS. Although the question of omission of radiotherapy was not addressed in a randomized fashion in HD15, the results suggest that omission of radiotherapy is safe in those with a negative end-of-treatment PET. In RATHL, patients with negative interim-PET were not recommended to undergo radiotherapy (unless the primary clinician believed that it was in the patient's best interest); only 6.5% of patients received consolidative radiotherapy compared with rates of 38% to 53% in previous studies. More recently, the GITIL study attempted to provide additional insight into whether radiotherapy could be omitted in certain patients by randomizing patients with a large nodal mass ≥5 cm and a negative end-of-treatment PET to no further therapy or 30 Gy consolidative radiotherapy. No significant difference was observed in the rate of long-term disease control (5-year PFS 97% vs 93% in RT vs no RT arms, respectively). These results suggest that, for most patients with advanced HL and negative PET at the conclusion of treatment, consolidative radiotherapy might be omitted without compromising the efficacy of treatment and sparing the long-term toxicities associated with this modality.

Taken together, these studies provide evidence that patients who demonstrate a response to frontline chemotherapy with a negative interim-PET might benefit from the decreased toxicity associated with reduced intensity chemotherapy and/or omission of consolidative radiotherapy without compromising the efficacy of frontline treatment. Both the NCCN[49] and ESMO[50] guidelines have incorporated the above findings. For example, both sets of guidelines recommend omission of bleomycin after the first 2 cycles of ABVD in patients with advanced HL and negative interim-PET. In addition, the ESMO guidelines recommend that patients who initially receive eBEACOPP and have a negative PET2 can safely complete a course of 4 cycles (rather than 6 cycles). Both sets of guidelines provide the option of omitting consolidative radiotherapy in patients with advanced disease and a negative end-of-treatment PET, although radiotherapy remains an option for those thought to be at high risk of relapse.

RESPONSE-ADAPTED THERAPY IN RELAPSED/ REFRACTORY HODGKIN LYMPHOMA

Only 1 study has investigated the use of PET-adapted salvage therapy in patients with relapsed or refractory (R/R) HL. Moskowitz and colleagues[71] enrolled 46 patients with R/R HL and all patients received 2 cycles of the anti-CD30 immunoconjugate, brentuximab vedotin (BV), as initial salvage therapy followed by PET. Patients who were PET-negative (DS 1–2) proceeded directly to high-dose chemotherapy (HDT) and ASCT, while those who had a positive PET after 2 cycles of BV went on to receive 2 cycles of ifosfamide, carboplatin, and etoposide (ICE), followed by HDT/ASCT in those who achieved PET negativity. Of 45 evaluable patients, 12 were PET-negative after BV alone and an additional 22 patients were PET-negative after ICE. Overall, 76% of patients achieved PET negativity and proceeded to HDT/ASCT per protocol. Similar rates of posttransplantation event-free survival were observed between those who received salvage with BV alone compared with those who received BV and ICE (92% and 91%, respectively). This compared with an event-free survival rate of 46% among those who were PET-positive after BV and ICE. This study provides evidence that a PET-adapted approach might be safe and feasible when used to select patients who might be candidates for less intensive salvage regimens.

CHALLENGES AND FUTURE PERSPECTIVES

At the same time that clinical investigators have been studying and refining response-adapted approaches to treatment in HL, the therapeutic armamentarium for HL has continued to expand. The anti-CD30 antibody-drug conjugate, BV, was the first novel agent to be approved for HL. Since the initial approval of this drug in 2011 for patients with relapsed/refractory HL, indications for its use have expanded, including as a frontline agent in combination with doxorubicin, vinblastine, and dacarbzine (A-AVD).[72] The prognostic significance of interim-PET scans is not well defined with this approach and NCCN guidelines recommend to continue A-AVD therapy in patients with DS 4 on interim imaging.

The programmed death-1 (PD-1) inhibitors, nivolumab and pembrolizumab, have also been approved for HL in the relapsed/refractory setting. Many trials investigating the role of these and other agents in the frontline setting have been completed or are ongoing. Currently, it is not clear how these drugs should be incorporated into response-adapted approaches to frontline treatment, although several trials are currently planned or underway that incorporate these novel agents into response-adapted protocols (NCT03517137, NCT02927769, or NCT03712202). One particular challenge that investigators will face when incorporating PD-1 inhibitors into trials of response-adapted treatment approaches is that of continued treatment beyond progression. Cohen and colleagues[73] reported on a single-arm, phase 2 study of nivolumab in patients with R/R HL, almost 30% of whom were treated beyond radiographic progression. Patients who had achieved at least stable disease as their best overall response to the prior line of therapy still derived significant clinical benefit and OS remained high. When using PD-1 inhibitors, a nuanced approach to defining response and treatment approach is warranted.

Although PET/CT has many strengths and is widely recognized as a standard assessment modality in HL, it is important to acknowledge that there are limitations to its use, which become apparent during the course of routine clinical practice. The use of PET/CT to predict clinical outcomes in HL must be accompanied by a recognition that this modality has imperfect sensitivity and specificity, which results in given false-negative and false-positive rates, respectively. Because the FDG molecule is not lymphoma-specific, but is taken up more efficiently into any glycolytically active cell, benign inflammation and infectious processes often appear FDG-avid on PET. A recent systematic review and meta-analysis on this topic found that more than 50% of positive interim or end-of-treatment PET/CT scans show no malignancy when the lesions are biopsied (ie, are falsely positive).[74] Conversely, PET/CT can yield false-negative results because of limitations in spatial resolution[75] or by decreased FDG-avidity of viable tumor tissue following antilymphoma treatment.[76] Among patients with negative interim-PET, approximately 5% to 10% of patients with early-stage HL and 10% to 20% of patients with advanced HL will ultimately experience disease progression (ie, false-negative results). One recent study reported

marked inter-observer variability and advocated for modifications to the current Deauville criteria.[62] These issues are the current challenges with the current technology. Tests with greater discrimination are needed to more accurately measure active disease and predict treatment response. Combining FDG-PET with molecular biomarkers, such as circulating tumor DNA, is likely to enhance the predictive value of response assessment and help to refine response-adapted treatment approaches. Other approaches including metabolic tumor volume and its prognostic impact in HL are being investigated[77,78] and may need to be incorporated into the treatment algorithms.

SUMMARY

Remarkable advances have been made in the treatment of HL over the last several decades, transforming the disease from a highly fatal malignancy to one that is curable in most patients. The development of highly effective combined modality treatment paradigms has resulted in a high rate of cure for early-stage and advanced-stage HL, but this success has led to a need to minimize the long-term toxicities of therapy without sacrificing the gains that have been made in efficacy. This need to balance long-term toxicity with therapeutic efficacy has been the driving force behind the development of response-adapted approaches. An expanding body of literature supports the safety and efficacy of a response-adapted approach, particularly in advanced HL. More extended long-term follow-up of several of the studies discussed in this review will provide additional insight into whether these approaches result in improved survival and/or reduce the risk of long-term toxicity. Despite the advantages of FDG-PET, more work remains to identify increasingly accurate methods of predicting treatment response. Advances in this area will likely come from continued refinements in PET technology and the addition of molecular monitoring, such as changes in circulating tumor DNA. Finally, as studies of novel agents for HL move from the relapsed/refractory to the frontline setting, the thoughtful incorporation of response-adapted protocols into trial design is important to achieving the best outcomes for our patients.

REFERENCES

1. Siegel RL, Miller KD, Jemal A. Cancer statistics, 2018. CA Cancer J Clin 2018;68(1):7–30.
2. NIH surveillance, epidemiology, and end results program. Cancer stat facts: Hodgkin lymphoma. National Institutes of Health surveillance,

epidemiology, and end results program. Available at: https://seer.cancer.gov/statfacts/html/hodg.html. Accessed December 5, 2018.

3. Bair SM, Mato A, Svoboda J. Immunotherapy for the treatment of Hodgkin lymphoma: an evolving paradigm. Clin Lymphoma Myeloma Leuk 2018;18(6): 1–12.

4. Küppers R, Engert A, Hansmann M-L. Hodgkin lymphoma. J Clin Invest 2012;122(10):3439–47.

5. Green MR, Monti S, Rodig SJ, et al. Integrative analysis reveals selective 9p24.1 amplification, increased PD-1 ligand expression, and further induction via JAK2 in nodular sclerosing Hodgkin lymphoma and primary mediastinal large B-cell lymphoma. Blood 2010;116(17): 3268–77.

6. Roemer MGM, Advani RH, Ligon AH, et al. PD-L1 and PD-L2 genetic alterations define classical Hodgkin lymphoma and predict outcome. J Clin Oncol 2016;34(23):2690–7.

7. Lamprecht B, Kreher S, Anagnostopoulos I, et al. Aberrant expression of the Th2 cytokine IL-21 in Hodgkin lymphoma cells regulates STAT3 signaling and attracts Treg cells via regulation of MIP-3. Blood 2008;112(8):3339–47.

8. Ma Y, Visser L, Blokzijl T, et al. The CD4+CD26− T-cell population in classical Hodgkin's lymphoma displays a distinctive regulatory T-cell profile. Lab Invest 2008;88(5):482–90.

9. Gandhi MK, Lambley E, Duraiswamy J, et al. Expression of LAG-3 by tumor-infiltrating lymphocytes is coincident with the suppression of latent membrane antigen-specific CD8+ T-cell function in Hodgkin lymphoma patients. Blood 2006;108(7): 2280–9.

10. Bonadonna G. Historical review of Hodgkin's disease. Br J Haematol 2000;110:504–11.

11. Jacobs EM, Peters FC, Luce JK, et al. Mechlorethamine HCl and cyclophosphamide in the treatment of Hodgkin's disease and the lymphomas. JAMA 1968;203(6):392–8.

12. Gordon LI, Hong F, Fisher RI, et al. Randomized phase III trial of ABVD versus Stanford V with or without radiation therapy in locally extensive and advanced-stage Hodgkin lymphoma: an intergroup study coordinated by the Eastern Cooperative Oncology Group (E2496). J Clin Oncol 2013;31(6): 684–91.

13. Engert A, Haverkamp H, Kobe C, et al. Reduced-intensity chemotherapy and PET-guided radiotherapy in patients with advanced stage Hodgkin's lymphoma (HD15 trial): a randomised, open-label, phase 3 non-inferiority trial. Lancet 2012;379(9828):1791–9.

14. Engert A, Plütschow A, Eich HT, et al. Reduced treatment intensity in patients with early-stage Hodgkin's lymphoma. N Engl J Med 2010;363(7):640–52.

15. Engert A, Diehl V, Franklin J, et al. Escalated-dose BEACOPP in the treatment of patients with advanced-stage Hodgkin's lymphoma: 10 years of follow-up of the GHSG HD9 study. J Clin Oncol 2009;27(27):4548–54.

16. Viviani S, Zinzani PL, Rambaldi A, et al. ABVD versus BEACOPP for Hodgkin's lymphoma when high-dose salvage is planned. N Engl J Med 2011; 365(3):203–12.

17. Radford J, Illidge T, Counsell N, et al. Results of a trial of PET-directed therapy for early-stage Hodgkin's lymphoma. N Engl J Med 2015;372(17): 1598–607.

18. Johnson P, Federico M, Kirkwood A, et al. Adapted treatment guided by interim-PET-CT scan in advanced Hodgkin's lymphoma. N Engl J Med 2016;374(25):2419–29.

19. Travis LB, Hill D, Dores GM, et al. Cumulative absolute breast cancer risk for young women treated for Hodgkin lymphoma. J Natl Cancer Inst 2005;97(19): 1428–37.

20. Moskowitz CS, Chou JF, Wolden SL, et al. Breast cancer after chest radiation therapy for childhood cancer. J Clin Oncol 2014;32(21):2217–23.

21. de Bruin ML, Sparidans J, van't Veer MB, et al. Breast cancer risk in female survivors of Hodgkin's lymphoma: lower risk after smaller radiation volumes. J Clin Oncol 2009;27(26):4239–46.

22. Omer B, Kadan-Lottick NS, Roberts KB, et al. Patterns of subsequent malignancies after Hodgkin lymphoma in children and adults. Br J Haematol 2012;158(5):615–25.

23. Franklin J, Pluetschow A, Paus M, et al. Second malignancy risk associated with treatment of Hodgkin's lymphoma: meta-analysis of the randomised trials. Ann Oncol 2006;17(12):1749–60.

24. van den Belt-Dusebout AW, Aleman BMP, Besseling G, et al. Roles of radiation dose and chemotherapy in the etiology of stomach cancer as a second malignancy. Int J Radiat Oncol Biol Phys 2009;75(5):1420–9.

25. Morton LM, Dores GM, Curtis RE, et al. Stomach cancer risk after treatment for Hodgkin lymphoma. J Clin Oncol 2013;31(27):3369–77.

26. Swerdlow AJ, Schoemaker MJ, Allerton R, et al. Lung cancer after Hodgkin's disease: a nested case-control study of the relation to treatment. J Clin Oncol 2001;19(6):1610–8.

27. Swerdlow AJ, Higgins CD, Smith P, et al. Second cancer risk after chemotherapy for Hodgkin's lymphoma: a collaborative British cohort study. J Clin Oncol 2011;29(31):4096–104.

28. Lorigan P, Radford J, Howell A, et al. Lung cancer after treatment for Hodgkin's lymphoma: a systematic review. Lancet Oncol 2005;6(10):773–9.

29. Koontz MZ, Horning SJ, Balise R, et al. Risk of therapy-related secondary leukemia in Hodgkin

lymphoma: the Stanford University experience over three generations of clinical trials. J Clin Oncol 2013;31(5):592–8.

30. Eichenauer DA, Thielen I, Haverkamp H, et al. Therapy-related acute myeloid leukemia and myelodysplastic syndromes in patients with Hodgkin lymphoma: a report from the German Hodgkin Study Group. Blood 2014;123(11):1658–64.

31. van Nimwegen FA, Schaapveld M, Cutter DJ, et al. Radiation dose-response relationship for risk of coronary heart disease in survivors of Hodgkin lymphoma. J Clin Oncol 2016;34(3):235–43.

32. Martin WG, Ristow KM, Habermann TM, et al. Bleomycin pulmonary toxicity has a negative impact on the outcome of patients with Hodgkin's lymphoma. J Clin Oncol 2005;23(30):7614–20.

33. Behringer K, Mueller H, Goergen H, et al. Gonadal function and fertility in survivors after Hodgkin lymphoma treatment within the German Hodgkin Study Group HD13 to HD15 trials. J Clin Oncol 2013;31(2):231–9.

34. Hodgson DC, Pintilie M, Gitterman L, et al. Fertility among female Hodgkin lymphoma survivors attempting pregnancy following ABVD chemotherapy. Hematol Oncol 2007;25(1):11–5.

35. Okada J, Yoshikawa K, Imazeki K, et al. The use of FDG-PET in the detection and management of malignant lymphoma: correlation of uptake with prognosis. J Nucl Med 1991;32(4):686–91.

36. Newman JS, Francis IR, Kaminski MS, et al. Imaging of lymphoma with PET with 2-[F-18]-fluoro-2-deoxy-D-glucose: correlation with CT. Radiology 1994;190(1):111–6.

37. Hutchings M, Mikhaeel NG, Fields PA, et al. Prognostic value of interim FDG-PET after two or three cycles of chemotherapy in Hodgkin lymphoma. Ann Oncol 2005;16(7):1160–8.

38. Hutchings M, Loft A, Hansen M, et al. FDG-PET after two cycles of chemotherapy predicts treatment failure and progression-free survival in Hodgkin lymphoma. Blood 2006;107(1):52–9.

39. Gallamini A, Hutchings M, Rigacci L, et al. Early interim 2-[18F]fluoro-2-deoxy-D-glucose positron emission tomography is prognostically superior to international prognostic score in advanced-stage Hodgkin's lymphoma: a report from a joint Italian-Danish study. J Clin Oncol 2007;25(24):3746–52.

40. Cerci JJ, Pracchia LF, Linardi CCG, et al. 18F-FDG PET after 2 cycles of ABVD predicts event-free survival in early and advanced Hodgkin lymphoma. J Nucl Med 2010;51(9):1337–43.

41. Juweid ME, Stroobants S, Hoekstra OS, et al. Use of positron emission tomography for response assessment of lymphoma: consensus of the Imaging Subcommittee of International Harmonization Project in Lymphoma. J Clin Oncol 2007;25(5):571–8.

42. Meignan M, Gallamini A, Haioun C. Report on the first international Workshop on interim-PET-scan in lymphoma. Leuk Lymphoma 2009;50(8):1257–60.

43. Cheson BD, Fisher RI, Barrington SF, et al. Recommendations for initial evaluation, staging, and response assessment of Hodgkin and non-Hodgkin lymphoma: the Lugano classification. J Clin Oncol 2014;32(27):3059–67.

44. Younes A, Hilden P, Coiffier B, et al. International Working Group consensus response evaluation criteria in lymphoma (RECIL 2017). Ann Oncol 2017;28(7):1436–47.

45. Raemaekers JMM, André MPE, Federico M, et al. Omitting radiotherapy in early positron emission tomography-negative stage I/II Hodgkin lymphoma is associated with an increased risk of early relapse: clinical results of the preplanned interim analysis of the randomized EORTC/LYSA/FIL H10 trial. J Clin Oncol 2014;32(12):1188–94.

46. André MPE, Girinsky T, Federico M, et al. Early positron emission tomography response-adapted treatment in stage I and II Hodgkin lymphoma: final results of the randomized EORTC/LYSA/FIL H10 trial. J Clin Oncol 2017;35(16):1786–94.

47. Fuchs M, Goergen H, Kobe C, et al. PET-guided treatment of early-stage favorable Hodgkin lymphoma: final results of the international, randomized phase 3 trial HD16 by the German Hodgkin study group. San Diego (CA): ASH; 2018. Available at: https://ash.confex.com/ash/2018/webprogram/Paper114519.html.

48. Straus DJ, Jung S-H, Pitcher B, et al. CALGB 50604: risk-adapted treatment of nonbulky early-stage Hodgkin lymphoma based on interim-PET. Blood 2018;132(10):1013–21.

49. National Comprehensive Cancer Network guidelines: Hodgkin lymphoma. National Comprehensive Cancer Network. 2018. Available at: https://www.nccn.org/professionals/physician_gls/pdf/hodgkins.pdf. Accessed December 12, 2018.

50. Eichenauer DA, Aleman BMP, André M, et al. Hodgkin lymphoma: ESMO clinical practice guidelines for diagnosis, treatment and follow-up. Ann Oncol 2018;29(Supplement_4):iv19–29.

51. Hoskin PJ, Lowry L, Horwich A, et al. Randomized comparison of the Stanford V regimen and ABVD in the treatment of advanced Hodgkin's lymphoma: United Kingdom National Cancer Research Institute lymphoma group study ISRCTN 64141244. J Clin Oncol 2009;27(32):5390–6.

52. Federico M, Luminari S, Iannitto E, et al. ABVD compared with BEACOPP compared with CEC for the initial treatment of patients with advanced Hodgkin's lymphoma: results from the HD2000 Gruppo Italiano per lo Studio dei Linfomi Trial. J Clin Oncol 2009;27(5):805–11.

53. Diehl V, Franklin J, Pfreundschuh M, et al. Standard and increased-dose BEACOPP chemotherapy compared with COPP-ABVD for advanced Hodgkin's disease. N Engl J Med 2003;348(24):2386–95.

54. Gallamini A, Tarella C, Viviani S, et al. Early chemotherapy intensification with escalated BEACOPP in patients with advanced-stage Hodgkin lymphoma with a positive interim positron emission tomography/computed tomography scan after two ABVD cycles: long-term results of the GITIL/FIL HD 0607 trial. J Clin Oncol 2018;36(5):454–62.

55. Press OW, Li H, Schöder H, et al. US Intergroup trial of response-adapted therapy for stage III to IV Hodgkin lymphoma using early interim fluorodeoxyglucose-positron emission tomography imaging: Southwest Oncology Group S0816. J Clin Oncol 2016;34(17):2020–7.

56. Ganesan P, Rajendranath R, Kannan K, et al. Phase II study of interim-PET-CT-guided response-adapted therapy in advanced Hodgkin's lymphoma. Ann Oncol 2015;26(6):1170–4.

57. Zinzani PL, Broccoli A, Gioia DM, et al. Interim positron emission tomography response-adapted therapy in advanced-stage Hodgkin lymphoma: final results of the phase II part of the HD0801 study. J Clin Oncol 2016;34(12):1376–85.

58. Casasnovas O, Brice P, Bouabdallah R, et al. Randomized phase III study comparing an early PET driven treatment de-escalation to a not PET-monitored strategy in patients with advanced stages Hodgkin lymphoma: final analysis of the AHL2011 LYSA study. J Clin Oncol 2018;36(15_suppl):7503.

59. Borchmann P, Goergen H, Kobe C, et al. PET-guided treatment in patients with advanced-stage Hodgkin's lymphoma (HD18): final results of an open-label, international, randomised phase 3 trial by the German Hodgkin Study Group. Lancet 2017;390(10114):2790–802.

60. Biggi A, Gallamini A, Chauvie S, et al. International validation study for interim-PET in ABVD-treated, advanced-stage Hodgkin lymphoma: interpretation criteria and concordance rate among reviewers. J Nucl Med 2013;54(5):683–90.

61. Stephens D, Li H, Schöder H, et al. Long-term follow-up of SWOG S0816: response-adapted therapy for stage III/IV Hodgkin lymphoma demonstrates limitations of PET-adapted approach. San Diego (CA): ASH; 2018. Available at: https://ash.confex.com/ash/2018/webprogram/Paper113034.html.

62. Kluge R, Chavdarova L, Hoffmann M, et al. Inter-reader reliability of early FDG-PET/CT response assessment using the Deauville scale after 2 cycles of intensive chemotherapy (OEPA) in Hodgkin's lymphoma. PLoS One 2016;11(3):e0149072. Woloschak GE.

63. Aleman BMP, van den Belt-Dusebout AW, Klokman WJ, et al. Long-term cause-specific mortality of patients treated for Hodgkin's disease. J Clin Oncol 2003;21(18):3431–9.

64. van Leeuwen FE, Klokman WJ, Stovall M, et al. Roles of radiation dose, chemotherapy, and hormonal factors in breast cancer following Hodgkin's disease. J Natl Cancer Inst 2003;95(13):971–80.

65. Myrehaug S, Pintilie M, Tsang R, et al. Cardiac morbidity following modern treatment for Hodgkin lymphoma: supra-additive cardiotoxicity of doxorubicin and radiation therapy. Leuk Lymphoma 2008;49(8):1486–93.

66. Johnson PWM, Sydes MR, Hancock BW, et al. Consolidation radiotherapy in patients with advanced Hodgkin's lymphoma: survival data from the UKLG LY09 randomized controlled trial (ISRCTN97144519). J Clin Oncol 2010;28(20):3352–9.

67. Aleman BMP, Raemaekers JMM, Tirelli U, et al. Involved-field radiotherapy for advanced Hodgkin's lymphoma. N Engl J Med 2003;348(24):2396–406.

68. Ferme C, Sebban C, Hennequin C, et al. Comparison of chemotherapy to radiotherapy as consolidation of complete or good partial response after six cycles of chemotherapy for patients with advanced Hodgkin's disease: results of the groupe d'études des lymphomes de l'Adulte H89 trial. Blood 2000;95(7):2246–52.

69. Diehl V, Loeffler M, Pfreundschuh M, et al. Further chemotherapy versus low-dose involved-field radiotherapy as consolidation of complete remission after six cycles of alternating chemotherapy in patients with advance Hodgkin's disease. German Hodgkin Study Group (GHSG). Ann Oncol 1995;6(9):901–10.

70. Wiernik PH, Hong F, Glick JH, et al. Radiation therapy compared with chemotherapy for consolidation of chemotherapy-induced remission of advanced Hodgkin lymphoma: a study by the Eastern Cooperative Oncology Group (E1476) with >20 years follow-up. Leuk Lymphoma 2009;50(10):1632–41.

71. Moskowitz AJ, Schöder H, Yahalom J, et al. PET-adapted sequential salvage therapy with brentuximab vedotin followed by augmented ifosamide, carboplatin, and etoposide for patients with relapsed and refractory Hodgkin's lymphoma: a non-randomised, open-label, single-centre, phase 2 study. Lancet Oncol 2015;16(3):284–92.

72. Connors JM, Jurczak W, Straus DJ, et al. Brentuximab vedotin with chemotherapy for stage III or IV Hodgkin's lymphoma 2018;378(4):331–44.

73. Cohen JB, Engert A, Ansell SM, et al. Nivolumab treatment beyond investigator-assessed progression: outcomes in patients with relapsed/refractory classical Hodgkin lymphoma from the phase 2 checkmate 205 study. San Diego (CA): ASH; 2017.

Available at: http://www.bloodjournal.org/content/130/Suppl_1/650?sso-checked=true.

74. Adams HJA, Kwee TC. Controversies on the prognostic value of interim FDG-PET in advanced-stage Hodgkin lymphoma. Eur J Haematol 2016;97(6):491–8.

75. Kapoor V, McCook BM, Torok FS. An introduction to PET-CT imaging. Radiographics 2004;24(2):523–43.

76. Banning U, Barthel H, Mauz-Körholz C, et al. Effect of drug-induced cytotoxicity on glucose uptake in Hodgkin's lymphoma cells. Eur J Haematol 2006;77(2):102–8.

77. Kanoun S, Rossi C, Berriolo-Riedinger A, et al. Baseline metabolic tumour volume is an independent prognostic factor in Hodgkin lymphoma. Eur J Nucl Med Mol Imaging 2014;41(9):1735–43.

78. Moskowitz AJ, Schöder H, Gavane S, et al. Prognostic significance of baseline metabolic tumor volume in relapsed and refractory Hodgkin lymphoma. Blood 2017;130(20):2196–203.

PET with Fluorodeoxyglucose F 18/ Computed Tomography as a Staging Tool in Multiple Myeloma

Guldane Cengiz Seval, MD[a], Elgin Ozkan, MD[b], Meral Beksac, MD[a],*

KEYWORDS

• Multiple myeloma • Staging • PET/CT

KEY POINTS

- FDG PET/CT has been performed to stage patients with myeloma, to accurately evaluate response to therapy, and to detect the site of extramedullary disease and impinging relapse.
- FDG PET/CT has had potential prognostic value in staging, in the interim and at the end of treatment monitoring, and during follow-up.
- In recent years, various groups have reported very promising and concordant results with an overall sensitivity of 90% and specificity of 75%.
- It is important to note that MR imaging is still the gold standard as a highly sensitive test in the assessment of diffuse bone marrow involvement and cord compression.

INTRODUCTION

The classification and differential diagnosis of monoclonal gammopathies depends on clinical, biological, and radiologic criteria. However, it remains challenging in certain cases. Within these disorders, the most common is monoclonal gammopathy of undetermined significance (MGUS), which is asymptomatic and consistently precedes the development of multiple myeloma (MM).[1] Smoldering multiple myeloma (SMM) represents a midclinical stage between MGUS and MM. SMM progresses to MM at a rate of approximately 10% per year over the first 5 years after the diagnosis. Progression decreases to 3% per year over the next 5 years and 1.5% per year

thereafter.[2] However, of importance is that these progression rates are influenced by the underlying cytogenetic risk factors.[2] MM is the most malignant form of these disorders, presenting with a wide spectrum of signs and symptoms.[1] In the past decade, novel treatment options have dramatically prolonged the survival of patients with myeloma regardless of age.

Osteolytic bone disease is one of the most common features of MM, and is present in up to 80% of patients at diagnosis.[3] For decades, conventional skeletal survey (CSS) has been the gold-standard imaging procedure for the detection of myeloma-related bone disease[3]; however, the new 2014 International Myeloma Working Group (IMWG) diagnostic criteria mandates more

The authors declare that they have no conflicts of interest relevant to the article submitted to 'PET Clinics'.
[a] Department of Hematology, Ankara University School of Medicine, Cebeci Research and Application Hospital, Mamak, Amkara 06590, Turkey; [b] Department of Nuclear Medicine, Ankara University School of Medicine, Cebeci Research and Application Hospital, Mamak, Ankara 06590, Turkey
* Corresponding author. Department of Hematology, Ankara University Medical School, Cebeci Hospital, Ankara 06220, Turkey.
E-mail address: meral.beksac@medicine.ankara.edu.tr

PET Clin 14 (2019) 369–381
https://doi.org/10.1016/j.cpet.2019.03.009
1556-8598/19/© 2019 Elsevier Inc. All rights reserved.

sensitive cross-sectional imaging techniques for the diagnosis of MM.[4] In addition, the presence of myeloma-defining events is the main feature that discriminates MM from other plasma cell disorders. In 2015 the European Myeloma Network (EMN) proposed an imaging algorithm for use in myeloma-related bone disease and recommended whole-body, multidetector, low-dose computed tomography (WBLD-CT) for the detection of lytic lesions in myeloma (grade 1A). In asymptomatic patients with no lytic disease in WBLD-CT, whole-body MR imaging (or spine and pelvic MR imaging if whole-body MR imaging [WB-MR imaging] is not available) has to be performed and in the presence of 1 or more focal lesions are clarified as having symptomatic disease that needs therapy (grade 1A). PET in combination with computed tomography (PET/CT) is essential not only at diagnosis but also for response/progression assessment (grade 2B).[1] In 2017 the European Society for Medical Oncology (ESMO) designated WBLD-CT as the new standard for the diagnosis of lytic disease, MR imaging for the suspicion of spinal cord compression, and PET/CT for the evaluation of bone lesions according to availability and resources.[5] The EMN also recommends PET/CT for patients presenting with solitary plasmacytomas (SP) to rule out MM or multiple plasmacytoma.[6]

PET/CT using fluorine-18 (^{18}F)-fluorodeoxyglucose (FDG), a marker of glucose metabolism, has performance similar to that of morphologic imaging techniques in the detection of bone lesions. The blood glucose level must be measured before administering FDG. If the plasma glucose level is <11 mmol/L (or <200 mg/dL) the FDG PET/CT study can be performed, but if the plasma glucose level is ≥11 mmol/L (or ≥200 mg/dL) the imaging must be postponed or the patient excluded depending on the patient's circumstances and the trial being conducted. Insulin should not be used to reduce glucose levels (this leads to greater muscle uptake of FDG) unless the interval between administration of insulin and FDG is more than 4 hours.[7]

MR imaging is recommended in patients with SMM who are asymptomatic in order not to miss ≥1 nonequivocal focal bone lesion (FL) (diameter >5 mm) that changes the diagnosis from SMM to MM.[4,8] MR imaging specifies bone abnormalities in ≥90% of symptomatic patients with myeloma and seems to be the best procedure for assessing painful lesions and detecting medullary compression.[6] In patients with myeloma with equivocal FL in MR imaging, staging can be completed by a WBLD-CT or an FDG PET/CT to verify asymptomatic bone disease. On the other hand, in the post-treatment follow-up the MR images are less satisfactory because of the high frequency of false positivity, whereas FDG PET/CT seems to be more effective.[4,8]

This review comprises a comprehensive overview of FDG PET/CT imaging in combination with other convenient imaging procedures, with emphasis on post-therapy findings in patients with myeloma (**Figs. 1–4**).

PET WITH FLUORODEOXYGLUCOSE F 18/COMPUTED TOMOGRAPHY FOR MONOCLONAL GAMMOPATHY OF UNDETERMINED SIGNIFICANCE AND SMOLDERING MULTIPLE MYELOMA

According to the criteria established by the IMWG in 2003, patients with MGUS are defined by the presence of a serum protein spike (SPS) of <3 g/dL, a bone marrow plasmacytosis less than 10%, a normal free light chain ratio, and the lack of CRAB (increased calcium, renal failure, anemia, and bone lesions) features.[9] SMM is also characterized by the absence of CRAB, despite the occurrence of an SPS ≥3 g/dL with or without marrow plasmacytosis ≥10%.[9] Precursor conditions do not require a specific treatment, with the exception of high-risk SMM, which has t(4;14), del(17p), and gain (1q) risk of progression to overt MM within 6 months.[2] Accumulating evidence shows that an increased bone marrow microvessel density or evolving type of SPS are associated with more frequent progression.[10,11] However, the identification of increased angiogenesis is an invasive and laborious condition, reflects a limited consideration of the marrow at a single site, and ensures a restricted anatomic picture rather than a whole-body functional metabolic evaluation that is a distinctive feature of FDG PET/CT.[12]

As expected, PET/CT is not sensitive enough to reflect areas of increased metabolic activity among patients with MGUS lacking any diffuse marrow abnormalities or FL.[13] Negative findings should be accepted as reliable predictors of stable MGUS.[14] Most of the patients with low-risk SMM are also negative on FDG PET/CT.[15] When even indistinct focal or diffuse abnormalities of FDG uptake are observed in this precursor status, a higher risk of progression should be suspected and followed up closely. Of note, several biomarkers (SPS level, percentage of bone marrow plasma cells, serum free light chain ratio, percentage of aberrant plasma cells, tumor genetic abnormalities, and FLs at MR imaging) have already been postulated to clarify subgroups of patients with SMM with the highest risk of progression to MM.[16] To the best of our knowledge, among imaging techniques FDG PET/CT is a reliable method

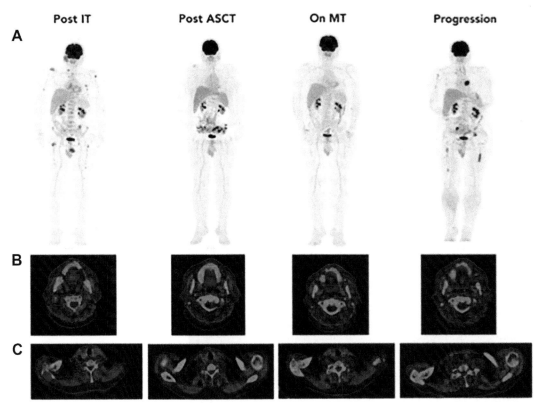

Fig. 1. A 63-year-old man with immunoglobulin G (IgG)-κ MM, ISS stage II, Durie-Salmon stage II. (*A*) MIP image, (*B*) and (*C*) transaxial fused PET/CT images. Post IT, response assessment after induction treatment; Post ASCT, response assessment after autologous stem cell transplantation; MT, response assessment during the maintenance treatment.

for evaluating early skeletal involvement and for predicting outcomes at the onset of MM.[17] In 2016 Zamagni and colleagues[18] reported the results of a prospective analysis of the prognostic implications of FLs as determined by FDG PEF/CT at the time of diagnosis in a group of patients with SMM (n = 120) who had been followed

without treatment. They observed that approximately 16% of the patients with SMM had a positive FDG PET/CT, mainly with a small number of FLs, and a low FDG uptake; a significantly higher risk of progression into overt MM occurred among these patients. On the basis of these results, integrating PET/CT scanning and axial MR imaging

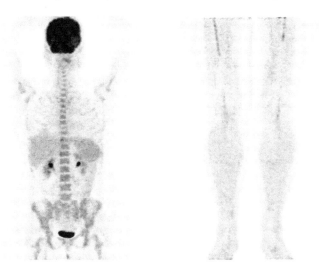

Fig. 2. A 42-year-old woman with IgM-κ restricted MM, ISS stage I, Durie-Salmon IIB. Whole-body ^{18}F-FDG PET/CT demonstrates diffuse homogeneous uptake of the bone marrow in the spine but also in the proximal limbs, and focal uptake in the bilateral proximal femur, suggesting diffuse bone marrow involvement associated with focal myeloma lesions.

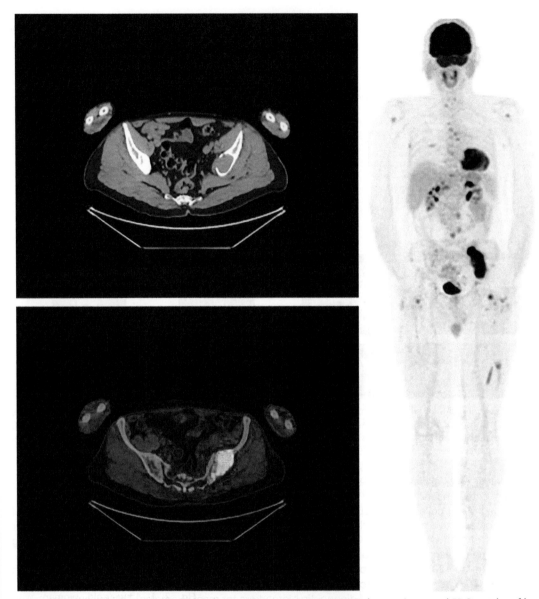

Fig. 3. A 62-year-old man with IgG-I MM, Durie-Salmon stage IIIA. PET/CT shows a increased FDG uptake of bone marrow that exceeds the liver uptake and a high-burden disease with a multi-focal pattern.

into the workup of patients with SMM may improve the management of the disease.

PET WITH FLUORODEOXYGLUCOSE F 18/ COMPUTED TOMOGRAPHY FOR MULTIPLE MYELOMA STAGING

In the Durie and Salmon myeloma staging system introduced in 1975, the detection of FLs by CSS correlated with measured myeloma cell mass.[19] This staging system has been widely used over the past 30 years. Unfortunately, despite low costs and wide employment and availability, the use of

conventional radiography, especially whole-body surveys, has several limitations. In light of these facts, Durie[20] introduced an update of their original staging system, the Durie-Salmon PLUS system, to improve the accuracy of anatomic and functional myeloma staging using advanced imaging modalities such as FDG PET/CT and MR imaging.

Durie and Barlogie were the first to notice the prognostic and diagnostic role of PET imaging at diagnosis. In 2002, Durie and colleagues[13] reported 16 patients with previously newly diagnosed MM (NDMM), 4 of whom (25%) had positive FDG PET/CT but negative conventional

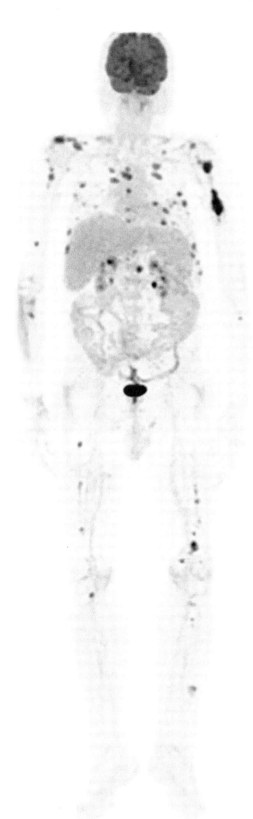

imaging. Four years later, Nanni and colleagues[21] conducted a study with 28 NDMM. They reported that PET/CT was able to determine a higher number of skeletal lesions than whole-body planar radiographs (WBPR) in 16 patients (57%), 9 of whom had a totally negative WBPR survey, whereas the 2 techniques detected roughly similar bony lesions in the remaining 12 patients (43%). When the results of PET/CT and MR imaging were compared, more positive findings with the former technique were seen in 25% of the patients and largely similar lesions with both techniques in 50%. On the contrary, MR imaging clarified particularly diffuse bone involvement and spine infiltration only, or more clearly. Despite its unchallenged usefulness, PET/CT cannot be accepted as the sole imaging procedure because this would result in the missed detection of small osteolyses and above all of diffuse spine and pelvis involvement.[22]

Following the demonstration of the role of FDG PET/CT in defining high-risk disease or follow-up of either patients with nonsecretory MM or those with complete response (CR), FDG PET/CT became a main part of myeloma studies in the United States. The National Oncologic PET Registry (NOPR), a large prospective program, included 22,975 patients with cancer in the first year and reported that 36.5% of the time, treating physicians modified the planned therapy because of PET/CT results.[23] NOPR has thus far enrolled over 1300 patients with myeloma. In a prospective study with 46 patients with NDMM; they compared the efficacy of FDG PET/CT, WBPR, and MR imaging. PET/CT was superior to WBPR in 46% of patients, including 19% with negative radiographs. However, in 30% of patients PET/CT imaging of the spine and pelvis failed to detect abnormal findings in areas in which MR imaging determined an abnormal pattern of bone marrow involvement, more frequently of diffuse type. In contrast, in 35% of patients PET/CT could detect the FL in areas that were out of the field of view of MR imaging. By performing MR imaging of the spine/pelvis and FDG PET/CT together, the ability to determine sites of medullary and extramedullary disease (EMD) was as high as 92%.[24]

Historically, the diagnosis of SP depends on biopsy-proven demonstration of localized monoclonal plasma cells (PCs) in a single lytic bone lesion or a soft-tissue mass. Localized disease in the absence of a systemic PC proliferative disorder accounts for less than 5% of all PC tumors.[25] More recently, a negative MR image of the spine and pelvis or no additional abnormal MR imaging evidence other than the single FL became recognized and requires confirmation of the diagnosis.

Fig. 4. A 54-year-old man with ISS stage I IgG-λ, Durie-Salmon IIIA. PET/CT shows a high degree of FDG avidity with a multifocal uptake pattern.

Depending on their location, 2 types of SP can develop: (1) solitary bone plasmacytoma (SBP); usually arising from the underlying bone through disruption of the cortical bone, over two-thirds of all SPs and generally involving vertebrae, femurs, ribs, and pelvis; (2) extramedullary plasmacytoma (EMP), which develops outside the bone marrow and within soft tissues, more frequently in the mucosa of the head and neck.[12,26] When diagnosing SP, the main drawbacks are (1) the possible coexistence of additional occult site(s) of the plasmacytomas not easily visualized by WBPR, and (2) the relative frequency of their progression into overt MM, consisting of approximately half of the patients with SBP and 30% of those with EMP within a decade.[12,26] Modern imaging techniques provide a major additive to the determination of occult lesions. In this setting, superiority of MR imaging of the axial skeleton has been demonstrated and is clearly recommended in patients with SBP of the spine and suspected cord or nerve root compression.[27,28] FDG PET/CT has provided negative or unclear findings in about 30% of the patients with MR imaging evidence of spine/pelvis involvement; a combination of anatomically limited MR imaging and metabolically sensitive FDG PET/CT would probably be required to obtain a comprehensive overview of both medullary and extramedullary sites of active MM.[24]

The incidence of single focal or multifocal EMD ranges in different series from 6% to 20% of patients with myeloma.[29] Usmani and colleagues[30] reported 936 patients with myeloma from a single center among whom those with EMD had a poor prognosis, including more commonly a genomically defined high-risk group in terms of shorter progression-free survival (PFS) and overall survival (OS). This observation underlines the importance of performing baseline FDG PET/CT imaging, which is crucial in evaluating the occurrence of EMD, known to be an independent prognostic factor in staging, in the interim and at final treatment monitoring, and during follow-up. In addition, PET/CT may result in a more targeted and individualized therapy. The main limitation of PET/CT is the lack of sensitivity in detecting diffuse bone marrow disease, whereas it is a highly sensitive technique in finding EMD. The sensitivity and specificity of PET/CT in occurrence of EMD is as high as 96% and 78%, respectively. Conversely, EMPs frequently develop in the head and neck area (nasal and paranasal cavities, oropharynx or nasopharynx, orbita, and larynx) and usually are not detected by MR imaging.[31]

In a systematic review and meta-analysis of 14 studies including almost 400 patients with myeloma, Lu and colleagues[32] concluded that FDG PET/CT is a reliable imaging technique with the highest dependability in terms of sensitivity, specificity, and positive and negative probability ratios for detecting intramedullary, but particularly extramedullary, sites of MM. In a retrospective analysis of 43 patients with a diagnosis of SP that depended on WBPR survey, the presence of ≥ 2 hypermetabolic lesions on FDG PET/CT and an abnormal serum free light chain ratio predict a rapid progression to MM.[33] In several studies of patients with a suspected diagnosis of SP, FDG PET/CT revealed occult osteolyses with or without soft-tissue masses that were not detectable by WBPR or MR imaging of the spine, in as much as 30% to 50% of cases.[27,34–36]

Various studies have demonstrated PET/CT as a dependable tool for most FL that are ≥ 1 cm in diameter using a maximum standardized uptake value (SUV_{max}) cutoff of 2.5 to indicate the presence of disease.[37] For lesions less than 5 mm in diameter, it has been recommended that any amount of FDG uptake should be accepted as positive regardless of SUV. Lesions between 5 and 10 mm are considered indeterminant if the SUV_{max} is less than 2.5. It is important to bear in mind that the patient's weight and body mass are additional factors that influence the SUV_{max}.[38]

Focal, multifocal, diffuse, and mixed patterns of FDG uptake are the standard demonstrations of MM on FDG PET/CT scan. No standard interpretation criteria have been established for the assessment of FDG PET/CT in plasma cell disorders. Some groups base their image interpretation mainly on semiquantitation; others have confidence in visual evaluation and others on both methods, which prevents repeatability.[39,40] In 2015, an Italian expert panel published Italian Myeloma criteria for PET use (IMPeTUs). Patients with myelom who had undergone FDG PET/CT at baseline (PET-0), after induction (PET-A1), and at the end of treatment (PET-EoT) were enrolled in this analysis (n = 17). At PET-0, the α coefficients for the bone marrow score, the score for the hottest FL, the number of FL, and the number of lytic lesions were 0.33, 0.47, 0.40, and 0.32, respectively. At PET-A1, the α coefficients were 0.09, 0.43, 0.22, and 0.21, respectively, and at PET-EoT the α coefficients were 0.07, 0.28, 0.25, and 0.21, respectively. Bone marrow was usually difficult to score because grades 2 and 3 are difficult to differentiate. However, because neither of the 2 grades is related to bone marrow myeloma involvement, the difference was not clinically significant. Based on all these results, the IMPeTUs criteria were found to be very helpful for clarifying the most critical points, and warrant prospective validation in a large cohort of patients with myeloma.[41]

COMPARATIVE ANALYSIS OF IMAGING TECHNIQUES IN THE MANAGEMENT OF PATIENTS WITH MYELOMA

Based on what has been discussed from the beginning of this review, it is clear that the introduction of the new functional imaging techniques has remarkably changed the approach to myeloma-related bone disease.[42] In 2009, the IMWG recommended that WBPR should remain the gold standard of the staging technique for both newly diagnosed and relapsed patients with myeloma. MR imaging or CT should be performed in patients with myeloma with clinically suspected bone disease but with normal conventional radiography and in those with apparent SP. In addition, MR imaging or CT should be urgently done when cord compression is suspected.[28] Of importance is that this consensus statement may not continue to be fully accepted. Despite the fact that conventional radiography has been the standard imaging technique for decades, a systematic review of the

more recent literature data has confirmed that the increasing use of MR imaging, CT, and FDG PET/CT provides a higher determination rate of myeloma-related bone disease in comparison with conventional imaging.[43] As expected, WBPR cannot be omitted when the presence of osteolyses of the skull and ribs is to be demonstrated. Even so, no conclusion can be drawn from this systematic review as to clear-cut superiority of one imaging modality at diagnosis or relapse. Nonetheless, it is thought that MR imaging and CT have equal diagnostic value, but MR imaging (unless contraindicated as a result of gadolinium intolerance, claustrophobia, metallic implants, or impaired renal function) does not involve exposure to radiation and should be preferred at diagnosis given its prognostic implications that are less clear and reliable with CT.[12] The strengths and weaknesses of all these imaging techniques in MM are shown in **Table 1** (data adapted from Mesguich and associates[44]).

Recently, FDG PET/CT has been used to stage patients with MM, to completely assess the response to treatment, to determine the site of EMD, and to assess relapse. It could represent diffuse involvement, FLs, or mixed bone disease

Table 1
Strength versus weakness of WBPR, WBCT, MR imaging, and PET/CT in multiple myeloma

	Strength	Weakness
WBPR	1. Large field of view 2. Lowest cost 3. Radiation < CT + PET/CT	1. Low sensitivity (particularly in early disease stage) 2. Imaging time > CT or PET/CT
WBCT	1. Sensitivity > WBPR 2. Fast whole-body exploration 3. Optimal for compression fractures instability characterization 4. Cost < MR imaging or PET/CT	1. Radiation > WBPR (1.3- to 3-fold) 2. Suboptimal for intramedullary lesions 3. Nonoptimal for assessing diffuse bone marrow involvement
MR imaging	1. Superior imaging modality for detection of diffuse bone marrow involvement 2. Sensitivity > WBPR or CT 3. Cost < PET/CT 4. No radiation 5. Optimal for brain and spinal cord imaging 6. Optimal for pathologic fracture characterization	1. Imaging time > WBPR or CT 2. Cost > WBPR or CT 3. Restricted field of view 4. Availability
PET/CT	1. Optimal for extramedullary disease assessment	1. Cost > WBPR, CT, MR imaging 2. Radiation > WBPR, CT, MR imaging 3. Suboptimal for diffuse bone marrow involvement and skull lesions 4. False positive at bone marrow biopsy site 5. Availability

From Mesguich C, Fardanesh R, Tanenbaum L, et al. State of the art imaging of multiple myeloma: comparative review of FDG PET/CT imaging in various clinical settings. Eur J Radiol 2014;83:2203–23.

with variable glucose uptake, resulting in heterogeneous SUV_{max}.

FDG PET/CT has some advantages in the evaluation of patients with myeloma[41]:

1. Extended field of view (including skull, ribs, upper limbs, femurs, pelvis, and spine)
2. Absence of possible collateral efficacy or adverse reactions to FDG
3. Possibility to conduct it even in patients with renal failure
4. Short image acquisition time with 3D tomographs (important in patients with fractures, bone pain, or vertebral collapse)
5. Free decubitus positioning
6. Possibility to assess soft tissues and organs at the same time to determine EMD
7. Probability to semiquantify disease activity using SUV_{max}
8. The low-dose CT images related to the PET/CT images allow the morphologic appearance of the bone to be clarified
9. No limitations in relation to metallic bone implants

However, FDG PET/CT imaging may be difficult to elucidate in some patients[41]:

1. A significant percentage of patients have MM-related anemia that results in a clear increment in bone marrow tracer uptake, causing a hot background in bone
2. The amount of FDG uptake is variable, hence a baseline study is warranted for reference
3. Early PET/CT-positive MM lesions may not cause an osteolytic area and may be difficult to clarify
4. The low spatial resolution of PET imaging does not present as "salt and pepper" bone marrow infiltration to be exactly determined
5. False-positive results may appear, especially in areas of inflammation or infection, deposits of brown fat (especially in the mediastinum and neck), recent fractures, postsurgical changes, vertebroplasty changes, and occasionally other benign or malignant processes, such as renal, pancreatic, uterine, and prostate cancer
6. Bone metallic implants may induce significant artifacts on CT images and may lead to infections with resulting nonspecific FDG uptake
7. Therapy response criteria are not identified

Limitations of conventional radiography led to routine incorporation of these imaging techniques into the diagnostic workup because of their higher sensitivity and ability to determine bone disease at an earlier phase than WBPR. The lower radiation exposure, lower cost, and higher availability mean that WBLD-CT is accepted as the gold-standard imaging for detecting lytic bone lesions in patients with with myeloma. PET/CT may be considered a precious option because it combines high sensitivity in identifying both lytic lesions (diameter of >5 mm) and extramedullary soft-tissue masses with the ability to provide reliable prognostic information.[45]

PROGNOSTIC VALUE OF PET WITH FLUORODEOXYGLUCOSE F 18 IN BASELINE EVALUATION

Bartel and colleagues[39] firstly compared the prognostic value of FDG PET and MR imaging in a large prospective trial comprising 239 patients with NDMM who received homogeneous first-line induction treatment consolidated with double autologous stem cell transplantation (ASCT). They reported that the number of FDG-avid FLs (>3) associated with the elevated levels of biological parameters (β2-microglobulin, C-reactive protein, and lactate dehydrogenase) indicated a poor prognosis, and that gene expression profiles were correlated with high-risk MM. In addition, the presence of greater than 3 FLs shortened PFS. Seven or more FLs at the baseline MR imaging correlated with a shorter event-free survival, but not OS. This finding was supported later in a study by Zamagni and colleagues[46] in a large series of 192 patients with myeloma treated with thalidomide-dexamethasone induction therapy and double ASCT, which demonstrated that ≥3 FLs (44% of cases), a SUV_{max} greater than 4.2 (46% of cases), and the presence of EMD (6%) had a negative impact on OS and PFS. Moreover, in the multivariate analysis the occurrence of EMD at diagnosis was correlated with a 5-fold higher risk of progression and mortality compared with patients without EMD. A smaller series of 61 patients (MM = 55 and SP = 6) also confirmed all the aforementioned findings, and only the presence of EMD with the highest SUV_{max} had an unfavorable prognostic value regarding OS in multivariate analysis ($P = .03$).[47]

An international collaboration led by Kostakoglu and colleagues[48] reporting PET results following induction before ASCT failed to prove the postinduction therapy IMWG and PET response to be independent prognosticators while the International Staging System (ISS) was a superior predictor. Another study comparing FDG PET and MR imaging in 33 patients with NDMM concluded that FDG PET had a prognostic value superior to MR imaging. The univariate and multivariate analysis demonstrated that FLs and diffuse bone marrow uptake on FDG PET shortened PFS ($P<.001$), whereas OS was affected only by the presence of FLs ($P = .001$). The MR imaging data were not predictive in multivariate analysis.[49]

Several studies also investigated the prognostic value of baseline volume-based FDG PET/CT parameters. These metrics, such as metabolic tumor volume (MTV) and total lesion glycolysis (TLG), are considered promising tools by quantifying functional disease burden in MM. In a study by McDonald and colleagues[50] with 192 patients with myeloma, baseline TLG greater than 620 g and MTV greater than 210 cm^3 were related to poor PFS and OS after adjusting for baseline myeloma variables. Combined with the 70-gene expression profiling (GEP 70) risk score, TLG >205 g defined a high-risk subgroup, and divided ISS stage II patients into 2 subgroups with outcomes similar to those of other ISS stages. However, depending on the heterogeneous data, further prospective clinical studies are warranted to confirm the validity of these results.

PET WITH FLUORODEOXYGLUCOSE F 18/ COMPUTED TOMOGRAPHY FOR THERAPEUTIC ASSESSMENT

Recommendations for PET/CT interpretation in patients with myeloma under treatment are summarized in **Table 2**.[44] The aforementioned study (Zamagni and colleagues[46]) reported that 35% of the patients still had positive FDG PET/CT imaging 3 months after ASCT. The clinical CR or very good partial response with negative PET/CT after a double ASCT was positively correlated with favorable PFS and OS. Likewise, patients achieving a CR but still having positive PET/CT imaging reportedly constituted a poor prognostic factor.

Finally, the French IMAJEM study was conducted in 134 patients with NDMM treated in the Intergroupe Francophone du Myelome/Dana-Farber Cancer Institute (IFM/DFCI) 2009 clinical trial. They aimed at comparing FDG PET/CT and MR imaging with respect to the detection of FLs at diagnosis, after 3 cycles of induction chemotherapy and before maintenance therapy, and the prognostic value of the imaging techniques. In contrast to MR imaging, normalization of FDG PET/CT after 3 cycles of induction and before maintenance was associated with better PFS and OS.[51]

General information gathered from all these results can be summarized as: (1) FDG PET/CT may be used as an important and reliable prognostic imaging procedure to predict long-term outcome in patients with myeloma both at diagnosis and following ASCT; (2) the presence of persistently increased tracer uptake after ASCT may verify critical reassessment of the ongoing treatment and the modification of the therapeutic approach.[12]

PET WITH FLUORODEOXYGLUCOSE F 18/ COMPUTED TOMPGRAPHY FOR DETECTION OF PROGRESSION

In the post-therapy setting, FDG PET/CT and WB-MR imaging have been investigated to define the remission status according to the IMWG uniform response criteria in patients with myeloma who had undergone ASCT. This study was conducted on 104 lesions detected in 21 out of 31 patients with myeloma following ASCT. Both imaging techniques were compared in terms of sensitivity, specificity, positive/negative predictive values, and overall outcome. Concordant results were revealed only in 15% of the lesions.[40] Based on the results of this study, FDG PET/CT should be preferred when assessing the remission status after ASCT.

The interest of post-ASCT FDG PET/CT (+3 months and every +6–12 months) has also been evaluated in a prospective cohort of 77 patients with myeloma. The patients were divided into group 1 (relapsed) and group 2 (no relapsed). In group 1, the time to relapse (TTR) was prolonged in patients with negative FDG PET/CT (27.6 vs 18 months; $P = .05$); additionally SUV$_{max}$ was also positively correlated with TTR in the positive FDG PET/CT cohort ($P<.01$). In group 2, 27 patients had negative FDG PET/CT and 13 patients had positive FDG PET/CT with stable SUV$_{max}$ value in the follow-up.[52]

In 2014, Lapa and colleagues[53] reported the prognostic role of FDG PET/CT in patients with myeloma relapse after autologous and/or allogeneic stem cell transplantation (n = 37). They found that the absence of FDG-avid foci was a prognostic factor associated with delay in relapse and OS ($P<.01$). On the other hand, the presence of greater than 10 FLs was correlated with prolonged duration of response ($P<.01$) and OS ($P<.05$). Shorter TTR was also associated with SUV$_{max}$ greater than 18.57 and the presence of EMD ($P = .037$ and $P = .049$, respectively). Moreover, PET/CT influenced treatment strategies in 30% of patients, more frequently revealing occult sites of EMD.[53] An additional series of 99 patients, of whom 73% underwent allogeneic stem cell transplantation, demonstrated the value of PET/CT in detecting sites of active disease at the time of relapse or progression, with an overall sensitivity of 80%.[54] Combination of PET/CT with biological parameters resulted in a 100% specificity predicting relapse or progression.[40] Results published by

Table 2
Recommendations for PET/CT interpretation in patients with myeloma

Patterns	Pretherapy PET/CT	Post-therapy PET/CT	Potential False-Positive Findings
Focal bone uptake	Positive: • FDG uptake > physiologic bone marrow uptake[a] and/or > physiologic liver uptake[b] with or without a corresponding CT finding	Positive: • Stable lytic lesion on CT, or new osteolytic lesion or no CT lesion with focal FDG uptake > physiologic liver uptake[b]	• Post-traumatic • Osteoporotic fracture (vertebral body, ribs, sacrum) • Stress fracture (femoral head) • Bone infarct (femoral head) • DJD and arthritis process (costochondral joints, shoulder grid) • Kyphoplasty, orthopedic devices
	Negative: • Uptake corresponding to arthritic changes in the joints, osteophytes, seen on CT images • Uptake at sites of kyphoplasty and prosthesis is usually negative but should be interpreted in the context of clinical information Equivocal: • Uptake in rib fractures and any other bone fractures with sclerotic changes on the CT study	Negative: • Uptake associated with a previously lytic CT lesion with development of a sclerotic rim with FDG uptake corresponding to the sclerotic change	
Diffuse bone marrow uptake	Positive: • Uptake in the axial and appendicular skeleton > liver uptake[c] Negative: • Uptake in the axial and appendicular skeleton ≤ liver uptake	Homogeneous uptake regardless of the intensity should be correlated with spine and pelvic MR imaging and laboratory data Positive heterogeneous uptake with grade exceeding that seen in the liver	Bone marrow stimulator injection <48 h before PET/CT[d]

[a] In lumbar spine and/or pelvis.
[b] No known liver disease. In cases with known liver disease, for example, cirrhosis physiologic bone marrow uptake in the healthy lumbar spine or pelvis (noninvolved by disease) should be used as the reference site.
[c] Regardless of this description for diffuse disease PET/CT is not a sensitive method and MR imaging correlation is recommended.
[d] Injection of colony stimulators is not a common practice in MM.
From Mesguich C, Fardanesh R, Tanenbaum L, et al. State of the art imaging of multiple myeloma: comparative review of FDG PET/CT imaging in various clinical settings. Eur J Radiol 2014;83:2203–23.

the authors[55] are also consistent with these earlier findings.

PET/COMPUTED TOMOGRAPHY USING OTHER RADIOPHARMACEUTICALS

Certain studies have underlined the diagnostic impact of new radiotracers in MM. The use of the radiolabeled amino acid carbon-11 (^{11}C)-methionine (MET) with PET/CT showed ^{11}C-MET-positive lesions in normal cancellous bone in the majority of 19 patients with myeloma, and in all patients with EMD. MET provided more accurate information on both intramedullary and extramedullary disease, and seemed to be superior to FDG in most of the patients with myeloma.[56]

In a pilot study, Cassou-Mounat and colleagues[57] reported the comparison of ^{18}F-fluorocholine (FCH), a metabolite incorporated into different phospholipids essential in the formation of cell membranes, and FDG for the detection of myeloma-related lesions in 21 patients at time of disease, relapse, and progression. In the 15 patients with apparent FLs, the on-site reader determined 72 FDG foci versus 127 FCH foci (+76%), and the blinded reader 69 FDG foci versus 121 FCH foci (+75%), both differences being significant. Based on these results, PET performed for suspected relapsing or progressive MM would find more lesions by using FCH rather than FDG.

Despite the potential theoretic value, discouraging results have been published regarding the efficiency of ^{18}F-NaF in the staging of MM. This radiotracer reflects bone remodeling and is an interesting imaging technique for bone malignancies. ^{18}F-NaF does not seem to add significant information to FDG PET in patients with myeloma at diagnosis and in relapse/refractory setting according to previous studies.[58,59]

Theranostic radiopharmaceuticals have also been applied in MM. Chemokine receptor 4 (CXCR4) is overexpressed in the monoclonal PCs, and Wester and colleagues[60] have successfully developed a radiolabeled CXCR4 ligand (^{68}Ga-pentixafor) for PET/CT imaging. Proof of concept for visualization of CXCR4 expression has recently been demonstrated in patients with MM. To transfer this targeting vector to a therapeutic scenario, derivatives of the compound allowing labeling with the β-particle emitters [177]Lu- or ^{90}Y-pentixather have been developed for therapeutic purposes.[61] Radiolabeled monoclonal antibodies with radionuclides such as ^{64}Cu or [89]Zr also have efficacy in selected patients before antibody-based treatments,[62] and the feasibility of immuno-PET with ^{64}Cu has been demonstrated in myeloma mouse models.[63]

SUMMARY

Recently, FDG PET/CT has been performed to stage patients with myeloma, to accurately evaluate response to therapy, to detect the site of EMD, and to assess impinging relapse. FDG PET/CT has been potential prognostic value in staging, in the interim and at the end of treatment monitoring, and during follow-up. In recent years, various groups have reported very promising and concordant results with an overall sensitivity of 90% and specificity of 75%. It is important to note that MR imaging is still the gold standard as a highly sensitive test in the assessment of diffuse bone marrow involvement and cord compression.

Similarly to the reading scheme for lymphomas, concerted efforts have been made to standardize a scoring system, such as the IMPETUS criteria, and response assessment for FDG PET/CT imaging in MM. As described in this review, various groups have reported promising and concordant results. Recent introduction of hybrid PET/MR imaging systems will be of considerable value in the assessment of MM, providing, morphologic and functional information.

REFERENCES

1. Kumar SK, Rajkumar V, Kyle RA, et al. Multiple myeloma. Nat Rev Dis Primers 2017;3:17046.
2. Rajkumar SV. Multiple myeloma: 2018 update on diagnosis, risk-stratification, and management. Am J Hematol 2018;93:1091–110.
3. Terpos E, Kleber M, Engelhardt M, et al. European Myeloma Network guidelines for the management of multiple myeloma-related complications. Haematologica 2015;100(10):1254–66.
4. Rajkumar SV, Dimopoulos MA, Palumbo A, et al. International Myeloma Working Group updated criteria for the diagnosis of multiple myeloma. Lancet Oncol 2014;15(12):538–48.
5. Moreu P, Miguel JS, Sonnevel P. Multiple myeloma: ESMO clinical practice guidelines for diagnosis, treatment and follow up. Ann Oncol 2017;28(4):52–61.
6. Caers J, Garderet L, Kortüm M, et al. An European Myeloma Network recommendation on tools for diagnosis and monitoring of multiple myeloma: what to use and when. Hematologica 2018;103(11):1772–84.
7. Boellaard R, Delgado-Bolton R, Oyen WJG, et al. FDG PET/CT: EANM procedure guidelines for tumour imaging version 2.0. Eur J Nucl Med Mol Imaging 2015;42:328–54.
8. Dimopoulos MA, Hillengass J, Usmani S, et al. Role of magnetic resonance imaging in the management of patients with multiple myeloma: a consensus statement. J Clin Oncol 2015;33:657–64.
9. International Myeloma Working Group. Criteria for the classification of monoclonal gammopathies, multiple myeloma and related disorders: a report of the International Myeloma Working Group. Br J Haematol 2003;121:749–57.
10. Vacca A, Ribatti D, Roncali L, et al. Bone marrow angiogenesis and progression in multiple myeloma. Br J Haematol 1994;87:503–8.
11. Rajkumar SV, Mesa RA, Fonseca R, et al. Bone marrow angiogenesis in 400 patients with monoclonal gammopathy of undetermined significance, multiple myeloma, and primary amyloidosis. Clin Cancer Res 2002;8:2210–6.

12. Dammacco F, Rubini G, Ferrari C, et al. ^{18}F-FDG PET/CT: a review of diagnostic and prognostic features in multiple myeloma and related disorders. Clin Exp Med 2015;15:1–18.

13. Durie BG, Waxman AD, D'Agnolo A, et al. Whole-body (18)F-FDG PET identifies high-risk myeloma. J Nucl Med 2002;43:1457–63.

14. Healy CF, Murray JG, Eustace SJ, et al. Multiple myeloma: a review of imaging features and radiological techniques. Bone Marrow Res 2011;2011: 583439.

15. Adam Z, Bolcak K, Stanicek J, et al. Fluorodeoxyglucose positron emission tomography in multiple myeloma, solitary plasmocytoma and monoclonal gammopathy of unknown significance. Neoplasma 2007;54:536–40.

16. Rajkumar V, Landgren O, Mateos MV. Smoldering multiple myeloma. Blood 2015;125:3059–75.

17. Zamagni E, Cavo M. The role of imaging techniques in the management of multiple myeloma. Br J Haematol 2012;159:499–513.

18. Zamagni E, Nanni C, Gay F, et al. ^{18}F-FDG PET/CT focal, but not osteolytic, lesions predict the progression of smoldering myeloma to active disease. Leukemia 2016;30:417–22.

19. Durie BGM, Salmon SE. A clinical staging system for multiple myeloma. Cancer 1975;36:842–54.

20. Durie BGM. The role of anatomic and functional staging in myeloma: description of Durie/Salmon plus staging system. Eur J Cancer 2006;42:1539–43.

21. Nanni C, Zamagni E, Farsad M, et al. Role of ^{18}F-FDG PET/CT in the assessment of bone involvement in newly diagnosed multiple myeloma: preliminary results. Eur J Nucl Med Mol Imaging 2006;33: 525–31.

22. Breyer RJ 3rd, Mulligan ME, Smith SE, et al. Comparison of imaging with FDG PET/CT with other imaging modalities in myeloma. Skeletal Radiol 2006; 35:632–40.

23. Hillner BE, Siegel BA, Shields AF, et al. Relationship between cancer type and impact of PET and PET/CT on intended management: findings of the National Oncologic PET Registry. J Nucl Med 2008;49: 1928–35.

24. Zamagni E, Nanni C, Patriarca F, et al. A prospective comparison of ^{18}F-fluorodeoxyglucose positron emission tomography-computed tomography, magnetic resonance imaging of the spine and pelvis and whole-body planar radiographs in the imaging assessment of bone disease in newly diagnosed multiple myeloma. Haematologica 2007;92(1):50–5.

25. Dimopoulos MA, Moulopoulos LA, Maniatis A, et al. Solitary plasmacytoma of bone and asymptomatic multiple myeloma. Blood 2000;96:2037–44.

26. Chargari C, Vennarini S, Servois V, et al. Place of modern imaging modalities for solitary plasmacytoma: toward improved primary staging and treatment monitoring. Crit Rev Oncol Hematol 2012;82:150–8.

27. Nanni C, Rubello D, Zamagni E, et al. ^{18}F-FDG PET/CT in myeloma with presumed solitary plasmocytoma of bone. In Vivo 2008;22:513–7.

28. Dimopoulos M, Terpos E, Comenzo RL, et al. International myeloma working group consensus statement and guide- lines regarding the current role of imaging techniques in the diagnosis and monitoring of multiple myeloma. Leukemia 2009;23:1545–56.

29. Weinstock M, Ghobrial IM. Extramedullary multiple myeloma. Leuk Lymphoma 2013;54:1135–41.

30. Usmani SZ, Heuck C, Mitchell A, et al. Extramedullary disease portends poor prognosis in multiple myeloma and is overrepresented in high-risk disease even in the era of novel agents. Haematologica 2012;97:1761–7.

31. Sasaki R, Yasuda K, Abe E, et al. Multi-institutional analysis of solitary extramedullary plasmacytoma of the head and neck treated with curative radiotherapy. Int J Radiat Oncol Biol Phys 2012;82: 626–34.

32. Lu YY, Chen JH, Lin WY, et al. FDG PET or PET/CT for detecting intramedullary and extramedullary lesions in multiple myeloma: a systematic review and meta-analysis. Clin Nucl Med 2012;37:833–7.

33. Fouquet G, Guidez S, Herbaux C, et al. Impact of initial FDG-PET/CT and serum-free light chain on transformation of conventionally defined solitary plasmacytoma to multiple myeloma. Clin Cancer Res 2014;20:3254–60, 2014.

34. Schirrmeister H, Buck AK, Bergmann L, et al. Positron emission tomography (PET) for staging of solitary plasmacytoma. Cancer Biother Radiopharm 2003;18:841–5.

35. Salaun PY, Gastinne T, Frampas E, et al. FDG-positron-emission tomography for staging and therapeutic assessment in patients with plasmacytoma. Haematologica 2008;93:1269–71.

36. Kim PJ, Hicks RJ, Wirth A, et al. Impact of ^{18}F-fluorodeoxyglucose positron emission tomography before and after definitive radiation therapy in patients with apparently solitary plasmacytoma. Int J Radiat Oncol Biol Phys 2009;74:740–6.

37. Nosa's-Garcia S, Moehler T, Wasser K, et al. Dynamic contrast-enhanced MRI for assessing the disease activity of multiple myeloma: a comparative study with histology and clinical markers. J Magn Reson Imaging 2005;22:154–62.

38. Larson SM, Erdi Y, Akhurst T, et al. Tumor treatment response based on visual and quantitative changes in global tumor glycolysis using PET/FDG imaging. The visual response score and the change in total lesion glycolysis. Clin Positron Imaging 1999;2: 159–71.

39. Bartel TB, Haessler J, Brown TLY, et al. F18-fluorodeoxyglucose positron emission tomography in the

context of other imaging techniques and prognostic factors in multiple myeloma. Blood 2009;114(10): 2068–76.

40. Derlin T, Peldschus K, Munster S, et al. Comparative diagnostic performance of ^{18}F-FDG PET/CT versus whole-body MRI for determination of remission status in multiple myeloma after stem cell transplantation. Eur Radiol 2013;23(2):570–8.

41. Nanni C, Zamagni E, Versari A, et al. Image interpretation criteria for FDG PET/CT in multiple myeloma: a new proposal from an Italian expert panel. IMPeTUs (Italian Myeloma criteria for PET Use). Eur J Nucl Med Mol Imaging 2016;43(3):414–21.

42. Walker RC, Brown TL, Jones-Jackson LB, et al. Imaging of multiple myeloma and related plasma cell dyscrasias. J Nucl Med 2012;53:1091–101.

43. Regelink JC, Minnema MC, Terpos E, et al. Comparison of modern and conventional imaging techniques in establishing multiple myeloma-related bone disease: a systematic review. Br J Haematol 2013;162:50–61.

44. Mesguich C, Fardanesh R, Tanenbaum L, et al. State of the art imaging of multiple myeloma: comparative review of FDG PET/CT imaging in various clinical settings. Eur J Radiol 2014;83:2203–23.

45. Zamagni E, Tacchetti P, Cavo M. Imaging in multiple myeloma: Which? When? Blood 2018. https://doi.org/10.1182/blood-2018-08-825356.

46. Zamagni E, Patriarca F, Nanni C, et al. Prognostic relevance of 18-F FDG PET/CT in newly diagnosed multiple myeloma patients treated with up-front autologous transplantation. Blood 2011;118(23): 5989–95.

47. Hazdenar R, Aki SZ, Akdemir OU, et al. Value of ^{18}F-fluorodeoxyglucose uptake in positron emission tomography/computed tomography in predicting survival in multiple myeloma. Eur J Nucl Med Mol Imaging 2011;38(6):1046–53.

48. Kostakoglu L, Dingli D, Beksac M. Prognostic value of post-induction PET/CT in untreated MM patients undergoing ASCT. J Clin Oncol 2017;30(15).

49. Fonti R, Pace L, Cerchione C, et al. ^{18}F-FDG PET/CT, ^{99m}Tc-MIBI, and MRI in the prediction of outcome of patients with multiple myeloma: a comparative study. Clin Nucl Med 2015;40:303–8.

50. McDonald JE, Kessler MM, Gardner MW, et al. Assessment of total lesion glycolysis by ^{18}F FDG PET/CT significantly improves prognostic value of GEP and ISS in myeloma. Clin Cancer Res 2016; 23(8):1981–7.

51. Moreau P, Attal M, Karlin L, et al. Prospective evaluation of MRI and PET-CT at diagnosis and before maintenance therapy in symptomatic patients with multiple myeloma included in the IFM/DFCI 2009 trial. Blood 2014;124:3359.

52. Nanni C, Zamagni E, Celli M, et al. The value of ^{18}F-FDG PET/CT after autologous stem cell transplantation (ASCT) in patients affected by multiple myeloma (MM): experience with 77 patients. Clin Nucl Med 2013;38:e74–9.

53. Lapa C, Lückerath K, Malzahn U, et al. [18]FDG-PET/CT for prognostic stratification of patients with multiple myeloma relapse after stem cell transplantation. Oncotarget 2014;5:7381–91.

54. Derlin T, Weber C, Habermann CR, et al. ^{18}F-FDG PET/CT for detection and localization of residual or recurrent disease in patients with multiple myeloma after stem cell transplantation. Eur J Nucl Med Mol Imaging 2012;39(3):493–500.

55. Beksac M, Gunduz M, Ozen M, et al. Impact of PET-CT response on survival parameters following autologous stem cell transplantation among patients with multiple myeloma: comparison of two cut-off values. Blood 2014;124:3983.

56. Lapa C, Knop S, Schreder M, et al. ^{11}C-Methionine-PET in multiple myeloma: correlation with clinical parameters and bone marrow involvement. Theranostics 2016;6(2):254–61.

57. Cassou-Mounat T, Balogova S, Nataf V, et al. ^{18}F-fluorocholine versus ^{18}F-fluorodeoxyglucose for PET/CT imaging in patients with suspected relapsing or progressive multiple myeloma: a pilot study. Eur J Nucl Med Mol Imaging 2016;43: 1995–2004.

58. Sachpekidis C, Goldschmidt H, Hose D, et al. PET/CT studies of multiple myeloma using ^{18}F-FDG and ^{18}F-NaF: comparison of distribution patterns and tracers' pharmacokinetics. Eur J Nucl Med Mol Imaging 2014;41:1343–53.

59. Sachpekidis C, Hillengass J, Goldschmidt H, et al. Treatment response evaluation with ^{18}F-FDG PET/CT and ^{18}F-NaF PET/CT in multiple myeloma patients undergoing high-dose chemotherapy and autologous stem cell transplantation. Eur J Nucl Med Mol Imaging 2017;44:50–62.

60. Wester HJ, Keller U, Schottelius M, et al. Disclosing the CXCR4 expression in lymphoproliferative diseases by targeted molecular imaging. Theranostics 2015;5:618–30.

61. Herrmann K, Schottelius M, Lapa C, et al. First-in-human experience of CXCR4-directed endoradiotherapy with [177]Lu- and ^{90}Y-labeled pentixather in advanced-stage multiple myeloma with Extensive intra- and extramedullary disease. J Nucl Med 2016;57:248–51.

62. Kraeber-Bodere F, Bailly C, Chérel M, et al. Immuno-PET to help stratify patients for targeted therapies and to improve drug development. Eur J Nucl Med Mol Imaging 2016;43:2166–8.

63. Halime Z, Frindel M, Camus N, et al. New synthesis of phenyl-isothiocyanate C-functionalised cyclams. Bioconjugation and ^{64}Cu phenotypic PET imaging studies of multiple myeloma with the te2a derivative. Org Biomol Chem 2015;13:11302–14.

Fluorodeoxyglucose-PET/ Computed Tomography as a Predictor of Prognosis in Multiple Myeloma

Cristina Nanni, MD[a], Elena Zamagni, MD, PhD[b],*

KEYWORDS

• Multiple myeloma • [18]F FDG-PE/CT • Extramedullary disease

KEY POINTS

• Fluorodeoxyglucose-PET/CT is a valuable predictor of outcomes in multiple myeloma patients in different settings.
• More robust data come from studies in newly diagnosed patients treated with autologous stem cell transplantation.
• The number of focal lesions and the presence of extramedullary disease are the most powerful prognostic factors.
• Unfavorable PET prognostic factors frequently correlate with adverse prognostic factors related to the burden or the biology of multiple myeloma.
• Standardization of the technique is ongoing.

INTRODUCTION

The role of imaging in the work-up of patients with multiple myeloma (MM) is aimed at allowing the recognition of both the effects of myeloma cells on the skeletal system and the eventual presence of extramedullary disease (EMD). Among several available procedures, fluorodeoxyglucose F 18 (^{18}F FDG)-PET/CT is recognized as one of the most effective in this field: it is a dual technique that blends the ability to identify bone destruction and lytic lesions with assessment of tumor burden and disease activity, in different areas of the bone marrow (BM) and of the cancellous and cortical bone.[1] This is of particular interest because BM plasma cell (PC) infiltration in MM is not homogeneous. There is now a rich literature proving its added value over standard diagnostic flow charts in terms of number of detected lesions, as several studies have reported a sensitivity and specificity over 80%.[2]

Objective advantages of this technique, particularly important in MM, are the extended field of view (which generally includes skull, ribs, upper limbs, femurs, pelvis, and spine)[3,4]; the absence of possible collateral effects or adverse reactions; the possibility of performing the procedure in patients with renal failure; the fast image acquisition time with 3-D/digital tomographs (this is important for patients with fractures, bone pain, or vertebral collapses) with a standardized procedure; the possibility of evaluating soft tissues and organs at the same time to detect EMD[5]; the possibility of semi-quantifying the disease activity by means of the maximum standardized uptake value (SUVmax) and, consequently, assessing therapy efficacy; no restrictions in cases of metallic bone implants; and the possibility of describing morphologic appearances of bones at low-dose CT, associated with PET images.[3,4] In this regard, the CT part of a PET/CT may be considered broadly comparable

[a] Metropolitan nuclear medicine, Azienda Ospedaliera-Universitaria di Bologna S. Orsola Malpighi, Bologna, Italy; [b] "Seràgnoli" Institute of Hematology, Bologna University School of Medicine, Bologna, Italy
* Corresponding author.
E-mail address: e.zamagni@unibo.it

PET Clin 14 (2019) 383–389
https://doi.org/10.1016/j.cpet.2019.03.005

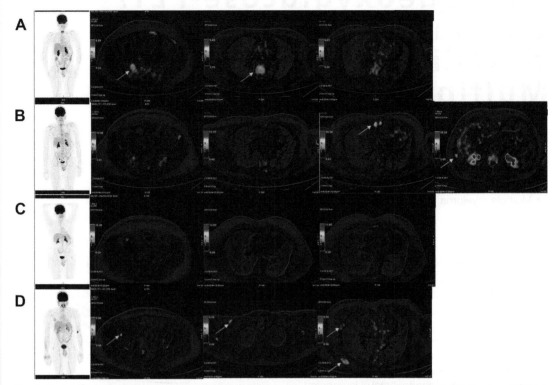

Fig. 1. Serial ^{18}F FDG-PET/CT in different phases of the disease in a patient affected by MM. (*A*) Staging. (*B*) Post-induction. (*C*) Post-ASCT/premaintenance. (*D*) At relapse. This case is an example of how much ^{18}F FDG-PET/CT provides prognostic parameters. This patient was studied at disease onset and had a positive PET. (*A*) On axial cuts of fused images, some bony FLs, as shown with the arrow (SUVmax 4.6). After induction (*B*), PET was normalized on these areas but some new lesions with high SUVmax (6 on the sternum) appeared, predicting a bad prognosis. After ASCT (*C*), a complete response was obtained but the patient experienced an early clinical relapse; at this moment, the PET scan was positive again (*D*) in a more extensive way.

to a whole-body low-dose CT, according to the minimum technical requirements established by the International Myeloma Working Group.[4] The ability to distinguish between metabolically active and inactive sites of MM renders fluorodeoxyglucose ^{18}F (FDG)-PET/CT an excellent tool to evaluate and monitor response to treatment. Despite morphologic stability of MM bone lesions, changes in metabolism (reflected in a modification of FDG uptake within lesions) are related to therapy effect and occur in a relatively short time. They can be easily measured both visually and semiquantitatively,[6] providing information on therapy efficacy, which is particularly helpful in nonsecretory MM (**Fig. 1**).

More recently, it also has been clearly demonstrated that the characteristics of PET involvement at diagnosis or during the course of the disease represent an important prognostic factor. MM is a heterogeneous disease. There is major variation in survival of MM patients, depending on several prognostic factors, related to patient characteristics (age, performance status, and comorbidities), tumor burden (assessed by the International

Staging System [ISS] and lactate dehydrogenase, intrinsic biology of the disease [cytogenetic abnormalities, circulating PCs, and EMD]), and response to therapy.[7] In this setting, new imaging techniques are assessing active MM at diagnosis (for staging and prognosis) and after treatment (for the evaluation of response), through morphologic and functional evaluations.

This review focuses on the role of ^{18}F FDG-PET/CT as predictor of prognosis in different MM settings.

FLUORODEOXYGLUCOSE-PET/COMPUTED TOMOGRAPHY AS PREDICTOR OF PROGNOSIS IN MULTIPLE MYELOMA
In Newly Diagnosed Transplant-eligible and Transplant-ineligible Patients

The independent impact of more than 3 focal lesions (FLs) at baseline and a PET involvement was frequently linked to adverse prognostic factors, such as high β_2-microglobulin, lactate dehydrogenase, C-reactive protein levels, and a high-risk gene expression profile (GEP), on shortened progression-free survival (PFS) and overall survival (OS) was first demonstrated in a series of patients treated upfront with novel agents and double autologous stem cell transplantation (ASCT).[8] In an updated report on the same series of patients, the number of FLs at ¹⁸F FDG-PET/CT (>3) and axial MR imaging (>7) was confirmed to be related to a high-risk GEP, which, in turn, was observed more frequently in patients with EMD.[9] Moreover, a comparison between GEP and whole-exome sequencing performed on paired random BM and FL aspirates showed different risk signatures, supporting the hypothesis that spatial clonal heterogeneity might contribute to disease progression.[10] In an independent series of patients prospectively treated with thalidomide-dexamethasone incorporated into double ASCT, the number of FLs (>3), the SUVmax value (>4.2), and presence of EMD at baseline were significantly related to shorter PFS and OS.[11] Of these parameters, both EMD and increased ¹⁸F FDG avidity retained independent prognostic relevance in a multivariate regression analysis. Several independent studies provided confirmatory results of the poor prognosis imparted by high ¹⁸F FDG uptake[12] and EMD that in turn was well detected by ¹⁸F FDG-PET/CT as part of the initial work-up.[13] The strong prognostic value of EMD detected at ¹⁸F FDG-PET/CT at baseline in terms of OS also was confirmed in a smaller series by a group from Turkish[14] as well as by the IMAgerie du JEune Myélome (IMAJEM) study,[15] reporting the poor prognostic value both of PET positive EMD at baseline on PFS and OS and of the presence of a high-risk cytogenetic profile (translocation t[4;14] and/or deletion del[17p] [$P = .004$]) on OS. Last study is particularly interesting because it provides a preliminary comparison between ¹⁸F FDG-PET/CT and MR imaging in terms of prognostic value. The endpoints were the detection of bone lesions at diagnosis by MR imaging versus PET/CT and the prognostic impact of MR imaging and PET/CT regarding PFS and OS. At diagnosis, MR imaging results were positive in 127 of 134 patients (95%), and PET/CT results were positive in 122 of 134 patients (91%; $P = .33$). Normalization of MR imaging after 3 cycles of RVD and before maintenance was not predictive of PFS or OS. PET/CT became normal after 3 cycles of RVD in 32% of the patients with a positive evaluation at baseline, and PFS was improved in this group (30-month PFS, 78.7% vs 56.8%, respectively). PET/CT normalization before maintenance was described in 62% of the patients who were positive at baseline. This was associated with better PFS and OS. EMD at diagnosis was an independent prognostic factor for PFS and OS, whereas PET/CT normalization before maintenance was an independent prognostic factor for PFS. Consistent with the findings reported in ASCT-eligible patients, the number of FLs, the SUVmax value, and EMD were strong predictors of adverse PFS and OS also in patients who were not candidates for ASCT.[16]

More complex PET biomarkers, such as functional volumes and tumor heterogeneity, also have been studied or are being evaluated with promising results. An initial pretherapeutic assessment of the metabolic tumor volume, whole-body (MTVWB) of FLs and EMD in 47 patients showed a poor prognostic value of high values on PFS and OS.[17] Another study on a series of 192 patients confirmed the poor prognostic value of a high MTVWB, which also was similar for a high total lesion glycolysis, whole body (TLGWB).[18] Combined with the GEP prognostic score (GEP70), a TLGWB greater than 205 g identified a high-risk subgroup and separated ISS II patients into 2 subgroups, with a similar outcome to ISS I and ISS III patients, respectively. The measurement of functional volumes, however, is not standardized at the moment and, therefore, although certainly prognostic, it is now not possible to report reproducible cutoffs.

Finally, Carlier and colleagues,[19] in the French IMAJEM study, reported that the presence of intratumoral textural features, reflecting tumor heterogeneity, seem to be another prognostic variable, derived by PET images. This is only a preliminary report, however, and more confirmatory studies are needed.

In Patients Receiving an Allogeneic Stem Cell Transplantation

The impact of ¹⁸F FDG-PET/CT on the outcomes of MM patients who received an allogenic stem cell transplantation (allo-SCT), either up-front or as salvage treatment, has been evaluated in a single study.[20] ¹⁸F FDG-PET/CT scans were performed within 30 days before allo-SCT and were positive in 59% of cases, revealing the presence of EMD in 11% and an SUVmax greater than 4.2 in 39%. In a multivariate regression analysis, EMD and high SUVmax were independent predictors of poor PFS and OS. Despite the retrospective nature of the analysis and the small number of patients, this study suggests that ¹⁸F FDG-PET/CT may be of help in predicting the outcomes of patients who are planned to receive an allo-SCT and provides the basis for the design of future prospective trials in this setting.

In Patients with Relapsed or Progressive Disease

In patients with MM and suspected relapse, a diagnosis requires direct indicators of tumor growth (at least 1 of the clone-related biomarkers)

Table 1
Studies of ^{18}F FDG-PET/CT as predictor of prognosis in patients with multiple myeloma

Reference	Study Design	No. of Patients	Parameter	Endpoint
At diagnosis, ASCT-eligible patients				
Bartel et al,[8] 2009	Prospective	239	FLs >3 vs ≤3	PFS: 66% vs 87% at 30 mo (P<.0001) OS: 73% vs 90% at 30 mo (P = .0002)
			EMD vs no EMD	PFS: 50% vs 82% at 30 mo (P<.0002) OS: 50% vs 87% at 30 mo (P<.002)
Zamagni et al,[11] 2011	Prospective	192	SUV >4.2 vs ≤4.2	PFS: 42% vs 66% at 4 y (P<.003) OS: 76% vs 92% at 4 y (P<.02)
			EMD vs no EMD	PFS: 22% vs 63% at 4 y (P<.000) OS: 64% vs 90% at 4 y (P<.02)
			FLs >3 vs ≤3	PFS: 50% vs 66% at 4 y (P<.006)
Haznedar et al,[14] 2011	Retrospective	61	EMD vs no EMD	OS: 62% vs n.r. at 5 y (P = .01)
McDonald et al,[18] 2017	Prospective	192	TLG, MTV	TLG >620 g and MTV >210 cm^3 remained prognostic factor of poor PFS and OS
At diagnosis, ASCT-ineligible patients				
Zamagni et al,[16] 2015	Retrospective	76	SUV >4.2, EMD and FLs >3	PFS: worst
Moreau et al,[15] 2017	Prospective	134	PET/CT vs MR imaging spine and pelvis at diagnosis	OS: worst Comparable
Prior to allo-ASCT				
Patriarca et al,[20] 2015	Retrospective	54	SUV >4·2 vs ≤4·2	PFS: 42% vs 72% at 2 y (P<.013) OS: 16% vs 51% at 2 y (P<.031)
			EMD vs no EMD	PFS: 50% vs 62% at 2 y (P<.016) OS: 12% vs 33% at 2 y (P<.010)
			FLs >1 vs ≤1	PFS: 49% vs 72% at 2 y (P<.075)
Premaintenance				
Moreau et al,[15] 2017	Prospective	134	Normalization of PET	OS: 21% vs 56% at 2 y (P<.033) PFS better in PET neg. 2-y OS rate of 94.2% vs 72.9%
			Normalization of MR imaging	Not predictive for PFS (P = .52) or OS (P = .62)
At relapse or progression				
Jamet et al,[25] 2019	Retrospective	40	FLs >6 in the app sk SUVmax >15.9	PFS (P = .01) OS (P = .04) PFS (P = .047)
Lapa et al,[22] 2014	Retrospective	37	FLs >10 vs ≤10	TTP: 4.1 vs 10.0 mo (P<.003) OS: 7.0 vs n.r. months (P<.023)
			EMD vs no EMD	TTP: 3.2 vs 29.3 mo (P<.049) OS: 8.8 vs n.r. months (P<.172)
Fonti et al,[17] 2012	Retrospective	47	< MTV	PFS: better OS: better

Abbreviations: app, appendicular; EMD, extra medullary disease; FLs, focal lesions; mo, months; MR magnetic resonance; MTV maximum tumor volume; N° number; neg, negative; n.r, not reached; OS, overall survival; PFS, progression free survival; sk, skeleton; SUV, standardized uptake volume; TLG, total lesion glycolisis; vs, versus; y, years;

and/or the presence of organ damage, including bone. PET/CT is of particular benefit if a biochemical progression is present, in disease with low tumor burden, or in patients who display a nonsecretory or oligosecretory phenotype at the time of disease progression, to provide an objective marker of disease activity in that situation.[21]

An analysis of the prognostic value of 18F FDG-PET/CT performed at the time of relapse or progression after prior ASCT or allo-SCT confirmed the favorable prognosis related to negative 18F FDG-PET/CT scans.[22] On the contrary, the number of FLs (>10), in particular those located in the appendicular skeleton, and EMD adversely affected both time to progression (TTP) and OS; shorter TTP also was associated with an SUVmax value greater than 18.5. 18F FDG-PET/CT findings influenced treatment strategies in 30% of patients, more frequently revealing occult sites of EMD. An additional study underscored the value of 18F FDG-PET/CT in detecting sites of active disease at the time of relapse/progression, with an overall sensitivity of 80%.[23] Combination of 18F FDG-PET/CT with laboratory data resulted in a 100% specificity in predicting relapse/progression.[18,24] In another study of patients in different MM phases, direct measurement of the tumor burden obtained by calculating the metabolic tumor volume (MTV) on 18F FDG-PET/CT images was used to predict PFS and OS.[17] Clinical outcomes for patients with an MTV below an identified cutoff were significantly better than those of patients with a value above the threshold value. These data, taken in aggregate, suggest that evaluation of metabolic activity provided by 18F FDG-PET/CT allows detecting relapse earlier, to distinguish between progressive and stable or nonviable MM and to confirm relapse/progression in equivocal cases, thus contributing to more careful identification of the prognosis of MM patients. Another recent study retrospectively analyzed the prognostic power of 18F FDG-PET/CT in 40 patients with a documented relapsing disease.[25] The investigators found that the presence of greater than 13 FLs and greater than 6 appendicular skeletal lesions and SUVmax greater than 15.9 predicted a shorter PFS, in contrast to ISS, high-risk cytogenetic abnormalities, and presence of EMD. The multivariate analysis confirmed the independent prognostic value of the presence of greater than 6 appendicular skeletal lesions and SUVmax greater than 15.9.

Available studies of 18F FDG-PET/CT as a determinant of prognosis in patients with newly diagnosed and relapsed/refractory MM are summarized in **Table 1**.

THE ISSUE OF INTERPRETATION

Due to possible interpretation issues and to the complexity of disease presentation and evolution, the need for standardization of PET reading is widely recognized. In literature, some groups based their image interpretation mainly on semi-quantitation, others on visual assessment, and others on both methods: all these aspects, unfortunately, prevents data reproducibility, especially in borderline cases and is an issue not only for routine image reading but also for the harmonization of results among different centers in multicenter trials. This acquires particular importance when PET is used for prognostication.

Mesguich and colleagues[26] proposed some indications to interpret MM 18F FDG-PET/CT in staging, interim evaluation, and after therapy. These indications, however, are not validated yet.

At the same time, a group of nuclear medicine experts, hematologists, and medical physicists defined new visual interpretation criteria (IMPeTUs) to standardize 18F FDG-PET/CT evaluation in MM patients. These include the visual interpretation of images based on the standard Deauville 5-point scale, taking into consideration different features of FDG distribution, such as the BM nonfocal uptake, focal bone lesions (site, number, and uptake), paramedullary lesions, and extramedullary lesions. These criteria currently are under perspective and multicenter European validation.[27] Other groups in Europe are proposing different interpretation criteria, partially corresponding to IMPeTUs[28] that also under validation. Total lesion glycolysis (TLG) and MTV are other methods proposed to assess the amount of active disease and its changes, as a consequence of therapy. TLG and MTV are 3-D regions of interest drawn taking into consideration standard measurement parameters, derived for all FLs with peak SUV above the background red marrow signal. There is not a standardized and widely accepted software, however, to harmonize these measurements in clinical practice, and much work is needed in the setting of clinical trials.

SUMMARY

18F FDG-PET/CT combines functional imaging provided by PET with morphologic evaluation assessed by CT, thus enabling detecting the presence of sites of metabolically active PCs, both inside and outside the BM, to define the anatomic localization, size, and metabolic properties of FLs and/or EMD, to predict patients' clinical outcomes, and to assess therapy-induced changes in tumor cell metabolism. Based on these attributes, ^{18}F FDG-PET/CT may be considered a valuable tool in the work-up of patients with newly diagnosed and relapsed/refractory MM, in particular for the detection of paramedullary and extramedullary soft tissue masses or solid organ involvement and for assessment of the risk imparted by the number of FLs and presence of EMD. Due to possible interpretation issues and complexity of disease presentation and evolution, the need for standardization of PET reading is widely recognized and currently ongoing.

REFERENCES

1. Zamagni E, Cavo M. The role of imaging techniques in the management of multiple myeloma. Br J Haematol 2012;159(5):499–513.
2. Nanni C, Zamagni E, Farsad M, et al. Role of 18F-FDG PET/CT in the assessment of bone involvement in newly diagnosed multiple myeloma: preliminary results. Eur J Nucl Med Mol Imaging 2006;33(5):525–31.
3. Van Lammeren-Venema D, Regelink JC, Riphagen II, et al. ^{18}F-fluoro-deoxyglucose positron emission tomography in assessment of myeloma-related bone disease: a systematic review. Cancer 2012;118(8):1971–81.
4. Cavo M, Terpos E, Nanni C, et al. Role of 18F-FDG positron emmission tomography/computed tomography in the diagnosis and management of multiple myeloma and other plasma cell dyscrasias: a consensus statement by the International Myeloma Working Group. Lancet Oncol 2017;18(4):e206–17.
5. Lu YY, Chen JH, Lin WY, et al. FDG PET or PET/CT for detecting intramedullary and extramedullary lesions in multiple Myeloma: a systematic review and meta-analysis. Clin Nucl Med 2012;37(9):833–7.
6. Boellaard R. Standards for PET image acquisition and quantitative data analysis. J Nucl Med 2009;50(Suppl 1):11S–20S.
7. Ziogas DC, Dimopoulous MA, Kastritis E. Progsnotic factors for multiple meyloma in the era of novel agents. Expert Rev Hematol 2018;11(11):863–79.
8. Bartel TB, Haessler J, Brown TL, et al. F18-fluorodeoxyglucose positron emission tomography in the context of other imaging techniques and prognostic factors in multiple myeloma. Blood 2009;114(10):2068–76.
9. Usmani SZ, Heuck C, Mitchell A, et al. Extramedullary disease portends poor prognosis in multiple myeloma and is over-represented in high-risk disease even in the era of novel agents. Haematologica 2012;97(11):1761–7.
10. Rasche L, Chavan SS, Stephens OW, et al. Spatial genomic heterogeneity in multiple myeloma revealed by multi-region sequencing. Nature Communication 2017. p. 1–11.
11. Zamagni E, Patriarca F, Nanni C, et al. Prognostic relevance of 18-F FDG PET/CT in newly diagnosed multiple myeloma patients treated with up-front autologous transplantation. Blood 2011;118(23):5989–95.
12. Park S, Lee SJ, Chang WJ, et al. Positive correlation between baseline PET or PET/CT findings and clinical parameters in multiple myeloma patients. Acta Haematol 2014;131(4):193–9.
13. Tirumani SH, Sakellis C, Jacene H, et al. Role of ^{18}F FDG-PET/CT in extramedullary multiple myeloma: correlation of ^{18}F FDG-PET/CT findings with clinical outcome. Clin Nucl Med 2016;41(1):e7–13.
14. Haznedar R, Aki SZ, Akdemir OU, et al. Value of 18F-fluorodeoxyglucose uptake in positron emission tomography/computed tomography in predicting survival in multiple myeloma. Eur J Nucl Med Mol Imaging 2011;38(6):1046–53.
15. Moreau P, Attal M, Caillot D, et al. Prospective evaluation of magnetic resonance imaging and [18F]fluorodeoxyglucose positron emission tomography-computed tomography at diagnosis and before maintenance therapy in symptomatic patients with multiple myeloma included in the IFM/DFCI 2009 trial: results of the IMAJEM study. J Clin Oncol 2017;35(25):2911–8.
16. Zamagni E, Nanni C, Mancuso K, et al. PET/CT improves the definition of complete response and allows to detect otherwise unidentifiable skeletal progression in multiple myeloma. Clin Cancer Res 2015;21(19):4384–90.
17. Fonti R, Larobina M, Del Vecchio S, et al. Metabolic tumor volume assessed by 18F-FDG PET/CT for the prediction of outcome in patients with multiple myeloma. J Nucl Med 2012;53(12):1829–35.
18. McDonald JE, Kessler MM, Gardner MW, et al. Assessment of total lesion glycolysis by 18F FDG PET/CT significantly improves prognostic value of GEP and ISS in myeloma. Clin Cancer Res 2017;23(8):1981–7.
19. Carlier T, Bailly C, Leforestier R, et al. Prognostic added value of PET Textural Features at diagnosis in symptomatic multiple myeloma. Oral communication SNM 201729.
20. Patriarca F, Carobolante F, Zamagni E, et al. The role of positron emission tomography with 18F-fluorodeoxyglucose integrated with computed tomography in the evaluation of patients with multiple myeloma undergoing allogeneic stem cell transplantation. Biol Blood Marrow Transplant 2015;21(6):1068–73.
21. Dupuis MM, Tuchman SA. Non-secretory multiple myeloma: from biology to clinical management. Onco Targets Ther 2016;9:7583–90.
22. Lapa C, Lückerath K, Malzahn U, et al. [18]F FDG-PET/CT for prognostic stratification of patients with multiple myeloma relapse after stem cell transplantation. Oncotarget 2014;5(17):7381–91.

23. Derlin T, Weber C, Habermann CR, et al. 18F-FDG PET/CT for detection and localization of residual or recurrent disease in patients with multiple myeloma after stem cell transplantation. Eur J Nucl Med Mol Imaging 2012;39(3):493–500.

24. Elliott BM, Peti S, Osman K, et al. Combining ¹⁸F FDG-PET/CT with laboratory data yields superior results for prediction of relapse in multiple myeloma. Eur J Haematol 2011;86(4):289–98.

25. Jamet B, Bailly C, Carlier T, et al. Added prognostic value of ¹⁸F FDG-PET/CT in relapsing multiple myeloma patients. Leuk Lymphoma 2019;60(1):222–5.

26. Mesguich C, Fardanesh R, Tanenbaum L, et al. State of the art imaging of multiple myeloma: comparative review of FDG PET/CT imaging in various clinical settings. Eur J Radiol 2014;83:2203–23.

27. Nanni C, Versari A, Chauvie S, et al. Interpretation criteria for ¹⁸F FDG-PET/CT in multiple myeloma (IMPeTUs): final results. IMPeTUs (Italian myeloma criteria for PET USe). Eur J Nucl Med Mol Imaging 2018;45(5):712–9.

28. Bodet-Milin C, Eugène T, Bailly C, et al. FDG-PET in the evaluation of myeloma in 2012. Diagn Interv Imaging 2013;94:184–9.

Fludeoxyglucose F 18 PET/Computed Tomography Evaluation of Therapeutic Response in Multiple Myeloma

Shaji Kumar, MD[a],*, Katrina N. Glazebrook, MD[b],
Stephen M. Broski, MD[b]

KEYWORDS

- Multiple myeloma • Response • Minimal residual disease • Extramedullary disease • PET • PET/CT

KEY POINTS

- Response assessment in myeloma primarily depends on measurement of monoclonal protein secreted by plasma cells, in the serum or urine.
- PET/computed tomography (CT) is useful in identifying both intramedullary and extramedullary disease in patients with multiple myeloma.
- Imaging can play a major role in response assessment in patients with myeloma with nonsecretory disease.
- Eradication of intramedullary myeloma without complete resolution of extramedullary disease may occur and hence sensitive, functional imaging studies such as PET/CT are required to confirm response of extramedullary disease.

BACKGROUND

Multiple myeloma (MM) is the second most common hematological malignancy after non-Hodgkin lymphoma and is characterized by the proliferation of terminally differentiated plasma cells (PCs), primarily in the bone marrow.[1–3] It is a disease of the older patient, with a median age at diagnosis of 67 years, and a male preponderance.[4] MM is always preceded by a precursor phase called monoclonal gammopathy of undetermined significance (MGUS), which is characterized by increased numbers of clonal plasma cells in the bone marrow without any associated end-organ damage or clinical signs or symptoms associated with the plasma cell proliferation.[5,6] Some patients may have an intermediate phase characterized by significant increase in the normal plasma cell burden but still without any appreciable end-organ damage,

referred to as smoldering MM (SMM).[7] Active MM is characterized by the presence of end-organ damage such as hypercalcemia, renal insufficiency, anemia, and destructive bone lesions, or markers of incipient disease progression such as high serum free light chain ratio (involved to uninvolved free light chain ratio $\geq$100), high proportion of PCs in the bone marrow ($\geq$60% PCs), or presence of more than 1 bone marrow lesion detected by MR imaging or PET/computed tomography (CT) scan.[8] Significant progress in MM treatment has occurred in the past decade with introduction of several effective therapies and use of multiple drugs in combination with autologous stem-cell transplantation (ASCT) in eligible patients. This, along with improved supportive care, has led to significant prolongation of survival in patients with MM.[9] However, MM remains incurable with current

[a] Division of Hematology, Mayo Clinic, 200 First Street Southwest, Rochester, MN 55905, USA; [b] Department of Radiology, Mayo Clinic, 200 First Street Southwest, Rochester, MN 55905, USA
* Corresponding author.
E-mail address: kumar.shaji@mayo.edu

PET Clin 14 (2019) 391–403
https://doi.org/10.1016/j.cpet.2019.03.006
1556-8598/19/© 2019 Elsevier Inc. All rights reserved.

treatment approaches and patients eventually become refractory to existing treatments and succumb to the disease.[10] Thus, there has been intense interest in developing novel therapeutic approaches that can achieve deep remissions in MM, improve long-term survival, and potentially provide a cure, or at minimum, chronic disease control with the help of sequential therapies.[11] This, in turn, has spurred interest in developing new methodologies for sensitive detection of minimal residual disease (MRD) in myeloma.

RESPONSE ASSESSMENT IN MYELOMA

The clonal PCs in MM predominantly reside in the bone marrow. Disease outside of the marrow presents as circulating PCs detectable by flow cytometry in most patients, and as extramedullary soft tissue disease in a smaller number of patients.[12–14] The clonal PCs in MM secrete monoclonal protein in the vast majority of patients and this can be measured in the serum or urine. Most patients, nearly 80%, secrete intact immunoglobulins that can be detected and measured by serum protein electrophoresis. This is most commonly an immunoglobulin (Ig)G, followed by an IgA immunoglobulin, with a smaller proportion of patients presenting with an IgD or IgM monoclonal protein. Serum immunofixation allows for identification of the monoclonal protein and detection of small amounts of monoclonal protein that cannot be identified on the serum protein electrophoresis. Approximately 15% of patients do not have an intact monoclonal immunoglobulin protein secreted by the clonal PCs, but rather have free kappa or lambda light chains unbound to a heavy chain. In most of these patients with light chain MM, the free immunoglobulin light chains are excreted into the urine and can be detected as Bence Jones proteins by urine protein electrophoresis. In a smaller number of patients, approximately 2% to 3%, the clonal PCs do not secrete any monoclonal protein, either in the form of intact immunoglobulins or free light chains and are termed as nonsecretory MM.[15] Although this situation is relatively uncommon in the setting of newly diagnosed MM (NDMM), over the course of disease evolution, the clonal PCs can become nonsecretory, resulting in an increasing proportion of patients with nonsecretory disease among those with relapsed and refractory myeloma.

Assessing response to treatment is an integral part of the management of any cancer and is particularly important for a disease like MM that is characterized by repeated remissions and relapses requiring frequent change in therapy. Response assessment and monitoring for disease relapse in MM has depended heavily on the measurement of the monoclonal protein in the serum and or urine using serum and urine protein electrophoresis, serum and urine immunofixation, and serum free light chain assay.[16] In patients with nonsecretory disease, the mainstay has been sequential measurement of bone marrow plasma cell content by aspiration, which can be quite cumbersome and traumatic for the patient. Up until now, the role of imaging has been limited to those patients in whom plasmacytomas had been identified before initiation of therapy. In these patients, serial imaging using radiographic skeletal surveys had been used for assessment of treatment response and monitoring of disease relapse. Given the inability of commonly used treatment approaches to achieve deep responses up until recently, there was no perceived need for very sensitive methods for detection of residual disease. However, with the introduction of multidrug combinations, especially in concert with high-dose chemotherapy and ASCT, complete response as defined by less than 5% PCs in the bone marrow and absence of monoclonal protein in the serum or urine on immunofixation has become much easier to achieve. This, in turn, highlighted the need to develop more sensitive methodologies to detect very small numbers of myeloma cells in the bone marrow. In recent years, 2 approaches have become mainstream for detection of MRD in MM, namely flow cytometry and next-generation sequencing. Both these technologies have the ability to detect 1 myeloma cell in 10^5 to 10^6 nucleated cells from the bone marrow aspirate. Prospective evaluation of MRD testing has demonstrated the importance of achieving MRD in prolonging progression-free (PFS) and overall survival (OS) in myeloma.[11,17–20] This has also highlighted the importance of detecting residual disease outside of the bone marrow to better define deep responses such as MRD negative status. In parallel with therapeutic advances, there has been significant progress in improving the sensitivity of various imaging modalities for detection of disease inside and outside of the bone marrow. This, in turn, has allowed the incorporation of imaging techniques such as PET/CT into the response assessment in MM. The current uniform response criteria from the International Myeloma Working Group (IMWG) is outlined in **Table 1**.[21]

ROLE OF IMAGING IN MYELOMA

Imaging has become increasingly important in diagnosis, prognostication, and assessment of therapeutic efficacy in MM and related disorders. More sensitive imaging approaches have made it

Table 1
International Myeloma Working Group diagnostic criteria for multiple myeloma

Disorder	Disease Definition
Non-immunoglobulin (Ig)M monoclonal gammopathy of undetermined significance (MGUS)	All 3 criteria must be met: • Serum monoclonal protein (non-IgM type) <3 g/dL • Clonal bone marrow plasma cells <10% • Absence of end-organ damage such as hypercalcemia, renal insufficiency, anemia, and bone lesions (CRAB) that can be attributed to the plasma cell proliferative disorder
IgM Monoclonal gammopathy of undetermined significance (IgM MGUS)	All 3 criteria must be met: • Serum IgM monoclonal protein <3 g/dL • Bone marrow lymphoplasmacytic infiltration <10% • No evidence of anemia, constitutional symptoms, hyperviscosity, lymphadenopathy, or hepatosplenomegaly that can be attributed to the underlying lymphoproliferative disorder
Light Chain MGUS	All criteria must be met: • Abnormal free light chain (FLC) ratio (<0.26 or >1.65) • Increased level of the appropriate involved light chain (increased kappa FLC in patients with ratio >1.65 and increased lambda FLC in patients with ratio <0.26) • No immunoglobulin heavy chain expression on immunofixation • Absence of end-organ damage that can be attributed to the plasma cell proliferative disorder • Clonal bone marrow plasma cells <10% • Urinary monoclonal protein <500 mg/24 h
Smoldering multiple myeloma	Both criteria must be met: • Serum monoclonal protein (IgG or IgA) $\geq$3 g/dL, or urinary monoclonal protein $\geq$500 mg per 24 h and/or clonal bone marrow plasma cells 10%–60% • Absence of myeloma defining events or amyloidosis

Multiple myeloma	Both criteria must be met:
	• Clonal bone marrow plasma cells $\geq$10% or biopsy-proven bony or extramedullary plasmacytoma
	• Any 1 or more of the following myeloma defining events:
	  ○ Evidence of end-organ damage that can be attributed to the underlying plasma cell proliferative disorder, specifically:
	    ■ Hypercalcemia: serum calcium >0.25 mmol/L (>1 mg/dL) higher than the upper limit of normal or >2.75 mmol/L (>11 mg/dL)
	    ■ Renal insufficiency: creatinine clearance <40 mL per minute or serum creatinine >177 μmol/L (>2 mg/dL)
	    ■ Anemia: hemoglobin value of >2 g/dL below the lower limit of normal, or a hemoglobin value <10 g/dL
	    ■ Bone lesions: 1 or more osteolytic lesions on skeletal radiography, computed tomography (CT), or PET/CT
	  ○ Clonal bone marrow plasma cell percentage $\geq$60%
	  ○ Involved: uninvolved serum FLC ratio $\geq$100 (involved FLC level must be $\geq$100 mg/L)
	  ○ >1 focal lesion on MR imaging studies (at least 5 mm in size)

Solitary plasmacytoma	All 4 criteria must be met: • Biopsy-proven solitary lesion of bone or soft tissue with evidence of clonal plasma cells • Normal bone marrow with no evidence of clonal plasma cells • Normal skeletal survey and MR imaging (or CT) of spine and pelvis (except for the primary solitary lesion) • Absence of CRAB

(continued on next page)

Table 1 (continued)	
Disorder	**Disease Definition**
Solitary plasmacytoma with minimal marrow involvement	All 4 criteria must be met: • Biopsy-proven solitary lesion of bone or soft tissue with evidence of clonal plasma cells • Clonal bone marrow plasma cells <10% • Normal skeletal survey and MR imaging (or CT) of spine and pelvis (except for the primary solitary lesion) • Absence of CRAB

clear that changes related to disease progression can be detected at a much earlier stage than previously possible with plain radiographs. This, along with studies demonstrating the ability of imaging to predict risk of disease progression in MM led to a revision of the myeloma diagnostic criteria to incorporate sensitive imaging studies such as MR imaging and PET/CT into the diagnostic algorithm.[8,22,23] The current IMWG diagnostic criteria are shown in **Table 2**. Use of advanced imaging has resulted in 2 critical changes in how we diagnose MM. Several studies have now shown that a PET/CT or low-dose whole-body CT scan can more sensitively identify presence of bone disease related to MM compared with radiographic skeletal survey.[24–26] Enhanced detection of osteolytic lesions results in many of the patients considered to have MGUS or SMM to be upstaged to active myeloma requiring therapy. In addition, MR imaging may detect bone marrow lesions that do not exhibit osteolysis on CT or radiograph, upstaging patients from precursor stages to active myeloma before bone destruction becomes visible. In addition to the current criteria for active MM that requires 2 or more bone marrow lesions, other aspects of these imaging modalities such as the pattern of bone involvement at baseline and evolving changes over time can predict increased risk of progression from SMM to active MM.[23]

In patients with active MM, advanced imaging modalities such as MR imaging and PET/CT can have prognostic value over and above their ability to confirm the diagnosis.[27,28] Routine use of these advanced imaging modalities can identify patients with extramedullary disease at the time of diagnosis (**Fig. 1**). Systematic use of imaging suggests that approximately 10% of patients with NDMM will have extramedullary disease at the time of initial diagnosis.[14] Patients with extramedullary disease appear to have an inferior outcome compared with patients in whom the disease is confined to the bone marrow. Specific patterns of bone marrow appearance on MR imaging of the spine, such as the diffuse pattern of involvement, have also been linked to differences in survival outcomes.

Another important contribution of imaging has been in assessing response to therapy in patients with MM. When imaging was limited to radiographs, the presence of lytic lesions was the typical abnormality that was identified at the time of diagnosis. However, these lesions do not change with treatment in the short term and cannot be used for assessing response to treatment, outside of disease progression, which can be indicated by increase in the number or size of the lesions. On the other hand, use of advanced imaging techniques, especially functional imaging, allows us to indirectly assess the degree of bone marrow infiltration and more importantly, the presence of disease outside of the bone marrow. This is particularly important, as disease within the bone marrow and in the extramedullary space can have differential response to therapy, and residual disease may be present at either site with complete disappearance from the other. Also, bone marrow aspiration may be falsely negative in some patients with patchy bone marrow involvement by malignant PCs. Prospective trials have demonstrated the additional value of imaging over conventional assessment of disease response using bone marrow examination and serum and urine monoclonal protein assessment.

ROLE OF PET/COMPUTED TOMOGRAPHY

Among the different modern imaging techniques in use today, PET/CT appears to be the most suited for the diagnosis, prognostication, and management of MM based on available data from both retrospective and prospective studies.[29–32] It can play an important role in the initial diagnostic assessment, as is evident from the current diagnostic criteria for active MM.[8] In addition to helping distinguish between SMM and active MM, PET/CT can also help differentiate solitary plasmacytoma from active MM.[33,34] In fact, a diagnosis of solitary plasmacytoma requires that additional foci of disease are definitively ruled out using a whole-body imaging modality such as PET/CT.[35] PET/CT also plays a very important role in the initial evaluation of nonsecretory disease.[36]

Table 2
International Myeloma Working Group uniform response criteria for multiple myeloma

Response Category	Response Criteria
Sustained minimal residual disease (MRD)	MRD negativity in the marrow (NGF or NGS, or both) and by imaging as defined below, confirmed minimum of 1 y apart. Subsequent evaluations can be used to further specify the duration of negativity (eg, MRD negative at 5 y)
Flow MRD	Absence of phenotypically aberrant clonal plasma cells by NGF on bone marrow aspirates using the EuroFlow standard operation procedure for MRD detection in multiple myeloma (or validated equivalent method) with a minimum sensitivity of 1 in 10^5 nucleated cells or higher
Sequencing MRD	Absence of clonal plasma cells by NGS on bone marrow aspirates in which presence of a clone is defined as fewer than 2 identical sequencing reads obtained after DNA sequencing of bone marrow aspirates using the LymphoSIGHT platform (or validated equivalent method) with a minimum sensitivity of 1 in 10^5 nucleated cells or higher
Imaging plus MRD	MRD negativity as defined by NGF or NGS plus disappearance of every area of increased tracer uptake found at baseline or a preceding PET/computed tomography (CT) or decrease to less than mediastinal blood pool standardized uptake value or decrease to less than that of surrounding normal tissue
Stringent complete response (sCR)	• CR as defined *plus* • Normal free light chain (FLC) ratio *and* • Absence of clonal PCs by immunohistochemistry or 2- to 4-color flow cytometry
Complete response (CR)	• Negative immunofixation of serum and urine *and* • Disappearance of any soft tissue plasmacytoma *and* • <5% plasma cells (PCs) in bone marrow *and* • If the only measurable disease is FLC, a normal FLC ratio
Very good partial response (VGPR)	• Serum and urine M-protein detectable by immunofixation but not on electrophoresis *or* • ≥90% reduction in serum M-protein and urine M-protein <100 mg/24 h • If the only measurable disease is FLC, a >90% reduction in the difference between involved and uninvolved FLC levels
Partial response (PR)	• If present at baseline, ≥50% reduction of serum M-protein and reduction in 24-h urinary M-protein by ≥90% or to <200 mg/24 h • If the only measurable disease is FLC, a ≥50% reduction in the difference between involved and uninvolved FLC levels • If the only measurable disease is BM, a ≥50% reduction in BM PCs (provided the baseline PCs was ≥30%) • If present at baseline, ≥50% reduction in the size (SPD) of soft tissue plasmacytomas
Minor response (MR)	• If present at baseline, ≥25% but ≤49% reduction of serum M-protein *and* reduction in 24-h urine M-protein by 50%–89% which still exceeds 200 mg/24 h *and* • If present at baseline, ≥50% reduction in the size (SPD) of soft tissue plasmacytoma
Stable disease (SD)	• Not meeting criteria for sCR, CR, VGPR, PR, MR or PD
Progressive disease (PD)	Increase of 25% from lowest value in any of the following: • Serum M-protein (absolute increase must be ≥0.5 g/dL) *and/or* • Urine M-protein (absolute increase must be ≥200 mg/24 h) *and/or* • If the only measurable disease is FLC, the difference between involved and uninvolved FLC levels (absolute increase must be >10 mg/dL) *and/or* • If the only measurable disease is BM, bone marrow PC percentage (absolute increase must be ≥10%)

(continued on next page)

Table 2 (continued)	
Response Category	**Response Criteria**
	Or any 1 or more of the following: • Development of new bone lesion or soft tissue plasmacytoma or ≥50% increase from nadir in the size (SPD) of existing bone lesions or soft tissue plasmacytoma or ≥50% increase in the longest diameter of a previous lesion >1 cm in short axis • 50% increase in circulating plasma cells (minimum of 200 cells/L) if this is the only measure of disease

Abbreviations: BM, bone marrow; NGF, next generation flowcytometry; NGS, next generation sequencing; SPD, sum of perpendicular diameters.

The pattern of PET/CT abnormalities seen in NDMM and relapsed myeloma can also have prognostic value.[30,37,38] Zamagni and colleagues[39] prospectively analyzed the prognostic relevance of PET/CT at diagnosis, after induction therapy, and ASCT in 192 patients with NDMM. Presence

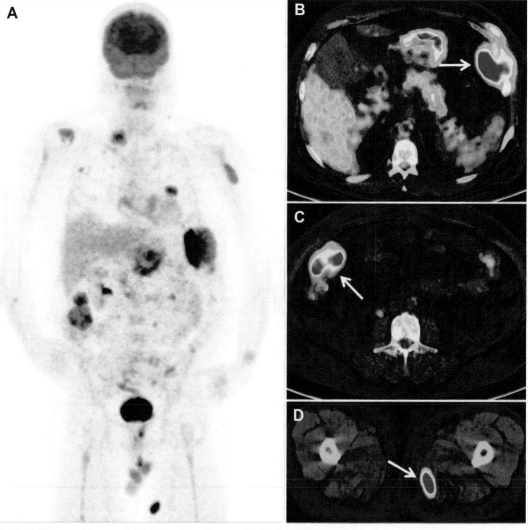

Fig. 1. A 53-year-old-man with MM undergoing staging FDG PET/CT. Maximum-intensity projection (*A*) and axial fused PET/CT images (*B–D*) demonstrate multiple sites of FDG avid extramedullary disease, including soft tissue extension of a lower left rib lesion (*arrow, B*), within the paracolic right lower quadrant (*arrow, C*), and within the soft tissues of the medial left thigh (*arrow, D*).

at baseline of at least 3 focal lesions (FLs) (44%), a standardized uptake value (SUV) >4.2 (46%), and extramedullary disease (6%) adversely affected PFS at 4 years (PFS; ≥3 FLs: 50%; SUV >4.2: 43%; presence of extramedullary disease (EMD): 28%). SUV greater than 4.2 and EMD were also correlated with shorter OS. Metabolic tumor volume measured using PET/CT may allow prediction of survival outcomes following therapy.[40]

However, among the most significant impact of PET/CT in the clinical management of MM has been in assessing response to treatment and detection of disease progression (**Figs. 2** and **3**). More recently, consensus criteria have been developed for use of PET/CT for disease assessment following therapy in MM. The Italian investigators have proposed the use of specific criteria for response assessment using PET (Italian Myeloma criteria for PET Use).[41]

PET/CT can play a unique role in assessing disease response in patients with solitary plasmacytoma, where serial PET/CT can be used to follow response to radiation therapy, both for demonstrating therapeutic effectiveness based on decreased fludeoxyglucose (FDG) activity in irradiated lesions, and also for monitoring local relapse and systemic progression.[42] In patients with extramedullary myeloma at the time of diagnosis or at the beginning of therapy for relapsed disease, it can be useful for serial monitoring of disease response.

In patients with nonsecretory disease, a PET/CT may be one of the few modalities to accurately assess disease response, and its noninvasive nature has benefits over performing multiple serial bone marrow aspirations. It can also be used monitor for relapse in these patients once treatment is completed. Even in patients with secretory disease, a combination of conventional paraprotein assessment and PET/CT may have better sensitivity in detection of disease progression.[43] Whether such early detection and intervention will alter the natural history of the disease remains unknown.

One of the areas in which PET/CT has particular utility is confirmation of MRD negativity following therapy in myeloma (see **Fig. 3**). Prospective studies have demonstrated that a negative PET/CT provides added value to bone marrow examination for residual PCs, again highlighting how the presence of extramedullary disease predicts outcomes in patients with myeloma.[44] The IFM group conducted a prospective comparison of MR imaging and PET/CT in patients with NDMM receiving a combination of lenalidomide, bortezomib, and dexamethasone (RVD) with or without ASCT, followed by lenalidomide maintenance in a phase 3 trial.[45] PET/CT and MR imaging were performed at diagnosis, after 3 cycles of RVD, and before maintenance therapy. At diagnosis, MR imaging was positive in 95%, and PET/CT was positive in 91% of patients. Normalization of MR imaging after 3 cycles of RVD and before maintenance was not predictive of PFS or OS. On the other hand, a negative PET/CT after 3 cycles of RVD was associated with improved PFS (30-month PFS, 78.7% vs 56.8%, respectively). In addition, maximal standardized uptake

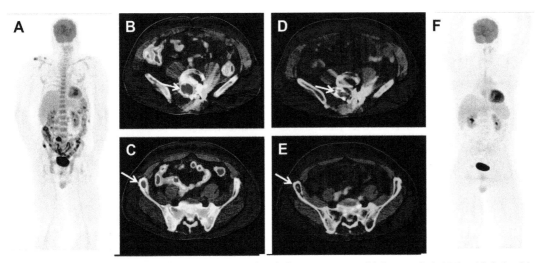

Fig. 2. A 55-year-old man with MM. Staging PET CT (*A–C*) demonstrates multiple osteolytic FDG avid skeletal lesions, including within the right L5 pedicle (*arrow, B*), and anterior right iliac wing (*arrow, C*). Restaging PET/CT after chemotherapy (*D–F*) demonstrates a complete metabolic response, with normalized activity in the right L5 pedicle (*arrow, D*) and anterior right iliac wing (*arrow, E*). Post-therapy FDG PET/CT confirmed negative bone marrow aspirate in this patient.

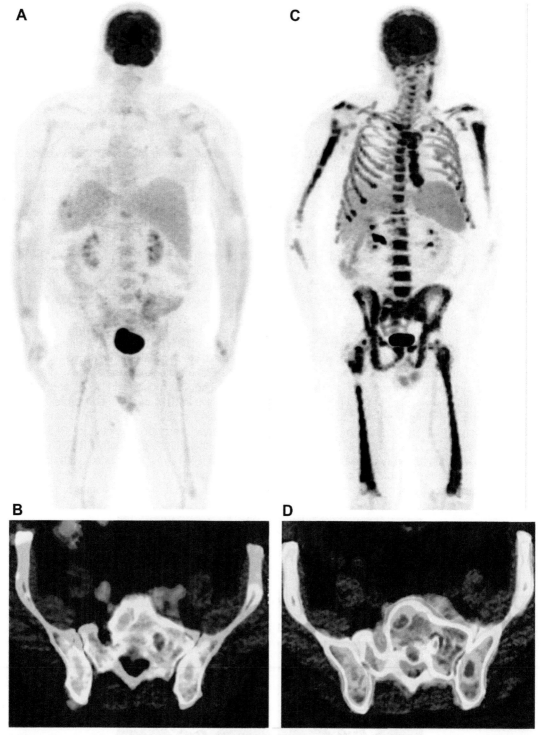

Fig. 3. A 51-year-old man with relapsed MM. Previous PET/CT (*A*, *B*) after chemotherapy and SCT demonstrated positive response, with near-normal FDG activity throughout the skeleton, including within multiple lytic lesions in the pelvis. Follow-up PET/CT (*C*, *D*) after laboratory evidence of disease relapse demonstrates new intense FDG activity throughout the marrow of the axial and proximal appendicular skeleton consistent with diffuse involvement by MM.

value reduction (Delta SUVmax) after 3 cycles was also predictive of improved PFS.[46] PET/CT normalization before maintenance was associated with better PFS and OS. The prognostic impact of a negative PET/CT was independent of the marrow MRD negativity, suggesting added value of imaging to marrow evaluation and paving the way for revision of the current IMWG response criteria.

PET/CT-based response appears to have an independent impact on survival outcomes, beyond the degree of response measured by conventional methods.[47] As part of Total Therapy 3 for NDMM, radiographic skeletal survey, MR imaging, and FDG PET/CT were evaluated in 239 untreated patients.[30] The number of FLs, especially those that were FDG avid on PET/CT correlated with other high-risk features. The presence of more than 3 FDG-avid FLs was an independent predictor of inferior OS and event-free survival. Complete FDG suppression in FLs before first transplantation conferred significantly better outcomes, independent of gene expression profiling-based risk assessment. In another study using tandem ASCT, persistence of SUV greater than 4.2 after induction was an early predictor for shorter PFS.[39] Three months after ASCT, patients with a negative PET/CT had superior 4-year PFS (89% vs 66%). In a multivariate analysis, both extramedullary disease and SUV greater than 4.2 at baseline and persistence of FDG uptake after ASCT were independent variables adversely affecting PFS. Similar data have also been seen in the context of allogeneic stem-cell transplantation (SCT) for myeloma.[48] Among 46 patients with evaluable PET/CT scans both before and 6 months after allogeneic SCT, the 23 patients who maintained or reached a PET complete remission showed a significantly prolonged PFS and OS compared with the 23 patients with persistence of any PET positivity (2-year PFS: 51% vs 25%, $P = .03$; 2-year OS: 81% vs 47%, $P = .001$).[49] Early evaluation using PET/CT after ASCT has been evaluated in the setting of Total Therapy, where more than 3 FLs on day 7 post-ASCT imparted inferior OS and PFS.[50] In contrast, the outcome of patients in whom the day 7 PET/CT demonstrated normalized FDG uptake appeared to be similar to those with fewer than 3 FLs at baseline.[51]

PET/CT has been compared with other imaging techniques for assessment of disease response, particularly whole-body MR imaging (WBMR imaging). In the posttreatment setting, both FDG PET/CT and WBMR imaging provide information about the extent of disease, allowing for more complete evaluation of persistent disease.

However, conventional MR imaging may be falsely positive because of persistent signal abnormality in treated, nonviable lesions.[52] This disadvantage of MR imaging may be overcome with the use of other techniques,[53] such as dynamic contrast-enhanced MR imaging and diffusion-weighted imaging.[54]

Although PET/CT has proven to be quite useful in initial disease staging and assessing response to treatment, it can certainly miss presence of disease, especially in the bone marrow.[55] Comparative studies suggest that MR imaging is more sensitive in detecting diffuse marrow infiltration with myeloma cells at baseline compared with PET/CT.[24,56–58] In addition, non-FDG avid myeloma from disease onset or at the time of relapse has also been reported. In some instances, this appears to be related to reduced expression of hexokinase-2, which has been shown to have lower expression in false-negative FDG PET/CT cases.[59] However, even in non-FDG avid disease, changes in the marrow attenuation on the low-dose CT portion of PET/CT can provide useful information regarding disease activity (**Fig. 4**).

NOVEL TRACERS FOR PET/COMPUTED TOMOGRAPHY

In addition to FDG, several other tracers have been studied in MM, with the hope that they may be more specific for detection of myeloma cells. For example, (11)C-methionine PET has been evaluated in patients with MM. In one study, all patients with MM except for one with purely extramedullary disease had (11)C-methionine-positive bone lesions. In contrast, control patients demonstrated homogeneous low uptake throughout the skeletal marrow.[60] Lesion and normal bone marrow (11) C-methionine mean SUVmax in patients with MM was 10.2 ± 3.5 and 4.3 ± 2.0, respectively, which were significantly higher than bone marrow uptake in the control group (mean SUVmax 1.8 ± 0.3; $P<.001$). Other studies have demonstrated relative advantages of (11)C-methionine versus FDG PET, including stronger correlation with biopsy-proven bone marrow involvement,[61] and higher sensitivity.[62] (11)C-acetate has been studied by several groups, and early data suggest that it may be more sensitive in identifying myeloma lesions, with added specificity compared with FDG PET.[63,64] L-[3-(18)F]-alpha-methyltyrosine ((18)F-FAMT) is a PET amino-acid tracer with uptake related to overexpression of L-type amino-acid transporter 1 and proliferative activity in tumor cells. In a small study of patients with MM, this radiotracer was found to be useful in detecting active myeloma lesions.[65]

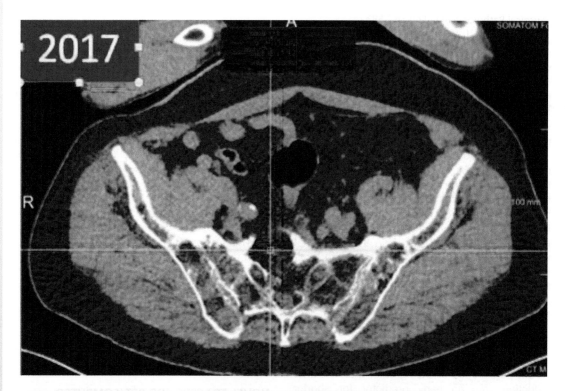

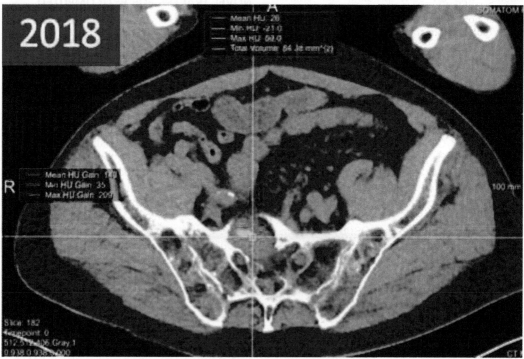

Fig. 4. A 76-year-old man diagnosed with MM in 2014, status post bone marrow transplantation in 2015. Whole-body low-dose CT from 2017 (*top*) shows a large lytic lesion in the upper sacrum with fatty marrow within the lesion (mean HU = −117). Follow-up CT scan in 2018 (*bottom*) demonstrates new soft tissue attenuation within the lesion (mean HU = 26) and a 143 HU mean increase in lesion attenuation consistent with disease relapse.

SUMMARY

PET/CT has become an integral part of myeloma management, including diagnosis, disease staging, prognostication, and most importantly, disease response assessment. It may be the best modality for response assessment in solitary plasmacytoma and nonsecretory disease and adds to bone marrow assessment in determining MRD status. Ongoing studies are exploring the feasibility of altering therapy based on short-term assessment of disease response using PET/CT, and novel PET radiotracers with potential advantages over FDG continue to be developed.

REFERENCES

1. Kumar SK, Rajkumar SV. The multiple myelomas - current concepts in cytogenetic classification and therapy. Nat Rev Clin Oncol 2018;15(7):409–21.
2. Kumar SK, Rajkumar V, Kyle RA, et al. Multiple myeloma. Nat Rev Dis Primers 2017;3:17046.
3. Siegel RL, Miller KD, Jemal A. Cancer statistics, 2018. CA Cancer J Clin 2018;68(1):7–30.
4. Kyle RA, Gertz MA, Witzig TE, et al. Review of 1027 patients with newly diagnosed multiple myeloma. Mayo Clin Proc 2003;78(1):21–33.
5. Kyle RA, Larson DR, Therneau TM, et al. Long-term follow-up of monoclonal gammopathy of undetermined significance. N Engl J Med 2018;378(3):241–9.
6. Landgren O, Kyle RA, Pfeiffer RM, et al. Monoclonal gammopathy of undetermined significance (MGUS) consistently precedes multiple myeloma: a prospective study. Blood 2009;113(22):5412–7.
7. Kyle RA, Remstein ED, Therneau TM, et al. Clinical course and prognosis of smoldering (asymptomatic) multiple myeloma. N Engl J Med 2007;356(25): 2582–90.
8. Rajkumar SV, Dimopoulos MA, Palumbo A, et al. International Myeloma Working Group updated criteria for the diagnosis of multiple myeloma. Lancet Oncol 2014;15(12):e538–48.
9. Kumar SK, Dispenzieri A, Lacy MQ, et al. Continued improvement in survival in multiple myeloma: changes in early mortality and outcomes in older patients. Leukemia 2014;28(5):1122–8.
10. Kumar SK, Lee JH, Lahuerta JJ, et al. Risk of progression and survival in multiple myeloma relapsing after therapy with IMiDs and bortezomib: a multicenter international myeloma working group study. Leukemia 2012;26(1):149–57.
11. Munshi NC, Avet-Loiseau H, Rawstron AC, et al. Association of minimal residual disease with superior survival outcomes in patients with multiple myeloma: a meta-analysis. JAMA Oncol 2017;3(1):28–35.
12. Paiva B, Paino T, Sayagues JM, et al. Detailed characterization of multiple myeloma circulating tumor cells shows unique phenotypic, cytogenetic, functional, and circadian distribution profile. Blood 2013; 122(22):3591–8.
13. Gonsalves WI, Rajkumar SV, Gupta V, et al. Quantification of clonal circulating plasma cells in newly diagnosed multiple myeloma: implications for redefining high-risk myeloma. Leukemia 2014;28(10): 2060–5.
14. Usmani SZ, Heuck C, Mitchell A, et al. Extramedullary disease portends poor prognosis in multiple myeloma and is over-represented in high-risk disease even in the era of novel agents. Haematologica 2012;97(11):1761–7.
15. Chawla SS, Kumar SK, Dispenzieri A, et al. Clinical course and prognosis of non-secretory multiple myeloma. Eur J Haematol 2015;95(1):57–64.
16. Durie BG, Harousseau JL, Miguel JS, et al. International uniform response criteria for multiple myeloma. Leukemia 2006;20(9):1467–73.
17. Yanamandra U, Kumar SK. Minimal residual disease analysis in myeloma - when, why and where. Leuk Lymphoma 2018;59(8):1772–84.
18. Anderson KC, Auclair D, Kelloff GJ, et al. The role of minimal residual disease testing in myeloma treatment selection and drug development: current value and future applications. Clin Cancer Res 2017; 23(15):3980–93.
19. Paiva B, Chandia M, Puig N, et al. The prognostic value of multiparameter flow cytometry minimal residual disease assessment in relapsed multiple myeloma. Haematologica 2015;100(2):e53–5.
20. Ladetto M, Ferrero S, Drandi D, et al. Prospective molecular monitoring of minimal residual disease after non-myeloablative allografting in newly diagnosed multiple myeloma. Leukemia 2016;30(5): 1211–4.
21. Kumar S, Paiva B, Anderson KC, et al. International Myeloma Working Group consensus criteria for response and minimal residual disease assessment in multiple myeloma. Lancet Oncol 2016;17(8): e328–46.
22. Kastritis E, Moulopoulos LA, Terpos E, et al. The prognostic importance of the presence of more than one focal lesion in spine MRI of patients with asymptomatic (smoldering) multiple myeloma. Leukemia 2014;28(12):2402–3.
23. Zamagni E, Nanni C, Gay F, et al. 18F-FDG PET/CT focal, but not osteolytic, lesions predict the progression of smoldering myeloma to active disease. Leukemia 2016;30(2):417–22.
24. Nanni C, Zamagni E, Farsad M, et al. Role of 18F-FDG PET/CT in the assessment of bone involvement in newly diagnosed multiple myeloma: preliminary results. Eur J Nucl Med Mol Imaging 2006; 33(5):525–31.
25. Hinge M, Andersen KT, Lund T, et al. Baseline bone involvement in multiple myeloma - a prospective

comparison of conventional X-ray, low-dose computed tomography, and 18flourodeoxyglucose positron emission tomography in previously untreated patients. Haematologica 2016;101(10):e415–8.

26. Dyrberg E, Hendel HW, Al-Farra G, et al. A prospective study comparing whole-body skeletal X-ray survey with 18F-FDG-PET/CT, 18F-NaF-PET/CT and whole-body MRI in the detection of bone lesions in multiple myeloma patients. Acta Radiol Open 2017;6(10). 2058460117738809.

27. Durie BG, Waxman AD, D'Agnolo A, et al. Whole-body (18)F-FDG PET identifies high-risk myeloma. J Nucl Med 2002;43(11):1457–63.

28. Durie BG. The role of anatomic and functional staging in myeloma: description of Durie/Salmon plus staging system. Eur J Cancer 2006;42(11): 1539–43.

29. Bredella MA, Steinbach L, Caputo G, et al. Value of FDG PET in the assessment of patients with multiple myeloma. AJR Am J Roentgenol 2005;184(4): 1199–204.

30. Bartel TB, Haessler J, Brown TL, et al. F18-fluoro-deoxyglucose positron emission tomography in the context of other imaging techniques and prognostic factors in multiple myeloma. Blood 2009;114(10): 2068–76.

31. Cavo M, Terpos E, Nanni C, et al. Role of (18)F-FDG PET/CT in the diagnosis and management of multiple myeloma and other plasma cell disorders: a consensus statement by the International Myeloma Working Group. Lancet Oncol 2017;18(4):e206–17.

32. Aljama MA, Sidiqi MH, Buadi FK, et al. Utility and prognostic value of (18) F-FDG positron emission tomography-computed tomography scans in patients with newly diagnosed multiple myeloma. Am J Hematol 2018;93(12):1518–23.

33. Siontis B, Kumar S, Dispenzieri A, et al. Positron emission tomography-computed tomography in the diagnostic evaluation of smoldering multiple myeloma: identification of patients needing therapy. Blood Cancer J 2015;5:e364.

34. Bhutani M, Turkbey B, Tan E, et al. Bone marrow abnormalities and early bone lesions in multiple myeloma and its precursor disease: a prospective study using functional and morphologic imaging. Leuk Lymphoma 2016;57(5):1114–21.

35. Nanni C, Rubello D, Zamagni E, et al. 18F-FDG PET/CT in myeloma with presumed solitary plasmocytoma of bone. In Vivo 2008;22(4):513–7.

36. Kaibara H, Kaida H, Ishibashi M, et al. 18F-FDG-PET findings of rare case of nonsecretory plasmablastic myeloma. Ann Nucl Med 2009;23(9):807–11.

37. Castellani M, Carletto M, Baldini L, et al. The prognostic value of F-18 fluorodeoxyglucose bone marrow uptake in patients with recent diagnosis of multiple myeloma: a comparative study with Tc-99m sestamibi. Clin Nucl Med 2010;35(1):1–5.

38. Haznedar R, Aki SZ, Akdemir OU, et al. Value of 18F-fluorodeoxyglucose uptake in positron emission tomography/computed tomography in predicting survival in multiple myeloma. Eur J Nucl Med Mol Imaging 2011;38(6):1046–53.

39. Zamagni E, Patriarca F, Nanni C, et al. Prognostic relevance of 18-F FDG PET/CT in newly diagnosed multiple myeloma patients treated with up-front autologous transplantation. Blood 2011;118(23):5989–95.

40. Fonti R, Larobina M, Del Vecchio S, et al. Metabolic tumor volume assessed by 18F-FDG PET/CT for the prediction of outcome in patients with multiple myeloma. J Nucl Med 2012;53(12):1829–35.

41. Nanni C, Versari A, Chauvie S, et al. Interpretation criteria for FDG PET/CT in multiple myeloma (IMPeTUs): final results. IMPeTUs (Italian myeloma criteria for PET USe). Eur J Nucl Med Mol Imaging 2018;45(5):712–9.

42. Adam Z, Bolcak K, Stanicek J, et al. Fluorodeoxyglucose positron emission tomography in multiple myeloma, solitary plasmocytoma and monoclonal gammapathy of unknown significance. Neoplasma 2007;54(6):536–40.

43. Elliott BM, Peti S, Osman K, et al. Combining FDG-PET/CT with laboratory data yields superior results for prediction of relapse in multiple myeloma. Eur J Haematol 2011;86(4):289–98.

44. Zamagni E, Nanni C, Mancuso K, et al. PET/CT improves the definition of complete response and allows to detect otherwise unidentifiable skeletal progression in multiple myeloma. Clin Cancer Res 2015;21(19):4384–90.

45. Moreau P, Attal M, Caillot D, et al. Prospective evaluation of magnetic resonance imaging and [(18)F]fluorodeoxyglucose positron emission tomography-computed tomography at diagnosis and before maintenance therapy in symptomatic patients with multiple myeloma included in the IFM/DFCI 2009 trial: results of the IMAJEM study. J Clin Oncol 2017;35(25):2911–8.

46. Bailly C, Carlier T, Jamet B, et al. Interim PET analysis in first-line therapy of multiple myeloma: prognostic value of DeltaSUVmax in the FDG-avid patients of the IMAJEM study. Clin Cancer Res 2018;24(21):5219–24.

47. Nanni C, Zamagni E, Celli M, et al. The value of 18F-FDG PET/CT after autologous stem cell transplantation (ASCT) in patients affected by multiple myeloma (MM): experience with 77 patients. Clin Nucl Med 2013;38(2):e74–9.

48. Stolzenburg A, Luckerath K, Samnick S, et al. Prognostic value of [(18)F]FDG-PET/CT in multiple myeloma patients before and after allogeneic hematopoietic cell transplantation. Eur J Nucl Med Mol Imaging 2018;45(10):1694–704.

49. Patriarca F, Carobolante F, Zamagni E, et al. The role of positron emission tomography with 18F-fluorodeoxyglucose integrated with computed tomography

in the evaluation of patients with multiple myeloma undergoing allogeneic stem cell transplantation. Biol Blood Marrow Transplant 2015;21(6):1068–73.

50. Usmani SZ, Mitchell A, Waheed S, et al. Prognostic implications of serial 18-fluoro-deoxyglucose emission tomography in multiple myeloma treated with total therapy 3. Blood 2013;121(10):1819–23.

51. Davies FE, Rosenthal A, Rasche L, et al. Treatment to suppression of focal lesions on positron emission tomography-computed tomography is a therapeutic goal in newly diagnosed multiple myeloma. Haematologica 2018;103(6):1047–53.

52. Derlin T, Peldschus K, Munster S, et al. Comparative diagnostic performance of (1)(8)F-FDG PET/CT versus whole-body MRI for determination of remission status in multiple myeloma after stem cell transplantation. Eur Radiol 2013;23(2):570–8.

53. Dutoit JC, Vanderkerken MA, Verstraete KL. Value of whole body MRI and dynamic contrast enhanced MRI in the diagnosis, follow-up and evaluation of disease activity and extent in multiple myeloma. Eur J Radiol 2013;82(9):1444–52.

54. Buemi F, Iannessi A, Carriero A, et al. Current concepts in tumor imaging with whole-body MRI with diffusion imaging (WB-MRI-DWI) in multiple myeloma and lymphoma AU - Stecco, Alessandro. Leuk Lymphoma 2018;59(11):2546–56.

55. Breyer RJ 3rd, Mulligan ME, Smith SE, et al. Comparison of imaging with FDG PET/CT with other imaging modalities in myeloma. Skeletal Radiol 2006;35(9):632–40.

56. Zamagni E, Nanni C, Patriarca F, et al. A prospective comparison of 18F-fluorodeoxyglucose positron emission tomography-computed tomography, magnetic resonance imaging and whole-body planar radiographs in the assessment of bone disease in newly diagnosed multiple myeloma. Haematologica 2007;92(1):50–5.

57. Hur J, Yoon CS, Ryu YH, et al. Comparative study of fluorodeoxyglucose positron emission tomography and magnetic resonance imaging for the detection of spinal bone marrow infiltration in untreated patients with multiple myeloma. Acta Radiol 2008;49(4):427–35.

58. Shortt CP, Gleeson TG, Breen KA, et al. Whole-body MRI versus PET in assessment of multiple myeloma disease activity. AJR Am J Roentgenol 2009;192(4):980–6.

59. Rasche L, Angtuaco E, McDonald JE, et al. Low expression of hexokinase-2 is associated with false-negative FDG-positron emission tomography in multiple myeloma. Blood 2017;130(1):30–4.

60. Dankerl A, Liebisch P, Glatting G, et al. Multiple myeloma: molecular imaging with 11C-methionine PET/CT–initial experience. Radiology 2007;242(2):498–508.

61. Lapa C, Knop S, Schreder M, et al. 11C-Methionine-PET in multiple myeloma: correlation with clinical parameters and bone marrow involvement. Theranostics 2016;6(2):254–61.

62. Nanni C, Zamagni E, Cavo M, et al. 11C-choline vs. 18F-FDG PET/CT in assessing bone involvement in patients with multiple myeloma. World J Surg Oncol 2007;5:68.

63. Ho CL, Chen S, Leung YL, et al. 11C-acetate PET/CT for metabolic characterization of multiple myeloma: a comparative study with 18F-FDG PET/CT. J Nucl Med 2014;55(5):749–52.

64. Lin C, Ho CL, Ng SH, et al. (11)C-acetate as a new biomarker for PET/CT in patients with multiple myeloma: initial staging and postinduction response assessment. Eur J Nucl Med Mol Imaging 2014;41(1):41–9.

65. Isoda A, Higuchi T, Nakano S, et al. (1)(8)F-FAMT in patients with multiple myeloma: clinical utility compared to (1)(8)F-FDG. Ann Nucl Med 2012;26(10):811–6.

PET/Computed Tomography in Chronic Lymphocytic Leukemia and Richter Transformation

Joanna M. Rhodes, MD[a],*, Anthony R. Mato, MD, MSCE[b]

KEYWORDS

- Chronic lymphocytic leukemia • Richter transformation • PET/CT • Accelerated CLL
- B-cell receptor inhibitor • Ibrutinib • Venetoclax

KEY POINTS

- PET/CT has a high negative predictive value for evaluating patients for Richter transformation.
- Choice of biopsy site to diagnose Richter transformation should be based on the maximum standardized uptake value (SUV_{max}), with SUV_{max} greater than or equal to 10 demonstrating the highest sensitivity and specificity in patients previously treated with chemoimmunotherapy. This cutoff may be less reliable in patients treated with B-cell receptor inhibitors due to its modestly lower sensitivity and specificity.
- The role of PET/CT to identify patients with high-risk chronic lymphocytic leukemia (without Richter transformation) has not been determined, and further studies are warranted in this area.

INTRODUCTION

Chronic lymphocytic leukemia (CLL) is the most common leukemia in the United States, and it is estimated that there will be 20,940 new cases in 2018.[1] CLL largely affects elderly patients, with median age of onset of 70.[1] CLL is defined as a neoplasm of small, mature B-lymphocytes that typically coexpress CD5, CD19, CD20(dim), and CD23.[2] A diagnosis of CLL is based on several features, including an absolute lymphocytosis of greater than or equal to 5×10^9 monoclonal B cells expressing the appropriate phenotype.[3]

Patients with CLL are clinically staged at diagnosis according to Rai staging and Binet staging, based on the degree of lymphocytosis, nodal involvement, splenomegaly, and blood counts (anemia and thrombocytopenia).[4–6] Asymptomatic patients are monitored closely under active observation.[2] Indications to initiate treatment include symptomatic lymphadenopathy, constitutional symptoms, cytopenias (including autoimmune related), and infectious complications related to an immunosuppressed state.[3] In addition to clinical staging, molecular and genetic markers have been identified for prognostication and to guide treatment choices. Two important markers that predict prognosis and treatment response are *TP53* interruption (17p deletion or TP3 mutation)[7–9] and immunoglobulin heavy chain variable (IGHV) somatic hypermutation.[10,11] Historically, chemoimmunotherapy (CIT) was recommended as first-line treatment.[12–15] The approval of B-cell receptor inhibitors (BCRis) and BCL2 inhibitors has

Disclosure Statement: J.M. Rhodes: None. A.R. Mato: COI: Consultancy: Abbvie, Celgene, Pharmacyclics, TG therapeutics, Acerta, Janssen, Sunesis, TG Therapeutics, Prime Oncology, and DAVA Oncology; Research Funding: Abbvie, Celgene, TG Therapeutics, Acerta, Janssen, Sunesis, and TG Therapeutics.
^a Division of Hematology and Oncology, Department of Medicine, Hospital of the University of Pennsylvania, Philadelphia, PA, USA; ^b CLL Program, Leukemia Service, Division of Hematological Oncology, Memorial Sloan Kettering Cancer Center, New York, NY, USA
* Corresponding author.
E-mail address: Joanna.rhodes@uphs.upenn.edu

PET Clin 14 (2019) 405–410
https://doi.org/10.1016/j.cpet.2019.03.007
1556-8598/19/© 2019 Elsevier Inc. All rights reserved.

revolutionized the treatment landscape and led to improvements in progression-free survival (PFS) and overall survival (OS) in all patients, particularly in patients with poor risk features.

CLL can undergo a Richter transformation (RT) to diffuse large B-cell lymphoma (DLBCL) or Hodgkin lymphoma (HL) in 1% to 10% of patients.[16–18] Despite recent therapeutic advances in CLL, there is no standard of care for RT management.[19–21] The prognosis remains poor, with a median OS estimated between 2.5 months and 10 months.[18,20,22–27] Additionally, several studies have demonstrated that RT outcomes are particularly poor in patients previously treated with BCRis.[25,26] Multiple risk factors for the development of RT have been identified, including mutations in *TP53*,[28] *NOTCH1*,[29] *SF3B1*,[30] B-cell receptor stereotype,[31] and complex karyotype.[32] Clinically, RT patients can present with B symptoms (fevers, chills, and night sweats), elevated lactate dehydrogenase (LDH), and rapidly progressive lymphadenopathy. Histologic diagnosis remains the gold standard and typically is achieved by either a core needle biopsy or excisional lymph node biopsy. Fine-needle aspiration is inadequate to diagnosis transformation of CLL.

PET/CT has been studied in the diagnosis and management of CLL and generally demonstrated minimal fludeoxyglucose F 18 (FDG) avidity[33,34] (**Fig. 1**). Recent studies have focused primarily on the use of PET/CT to identify sites for biopsy to confirm a clinical suspicion of RT as well as for CLL prognostication. The key question is whether PET/CT can distinguish CLL from histologic transformation.

PET/COMPUTED TOMOGRAPHY IN CHRONIC LYMPHOCYTIC LEUKEMIA

The first study to look exclusively at the role of PET/CT in the management of CLL was performed by Bruzzi and colleagues[33] (**Table 1**) In this single-center study, 26 patients with CLL were identified who underwent PET/CT as part of their routine care; 57 PET/CTs were performed, with each patient undergoing a mean of 2.5 scans (range 2–4). One scan was performed prior to treatment and 56 were performed in patients after therapy; 38 scans (in 18 patients) had a standardized uptake value (SUV) less than 5 and 19 had SUV greater than or equal to 5. Ten of 18 patients underwent tissue biopsy, which confirmed RT; 1 patient had HL; 3 patients had refractory CLL with extensive marrow involvement; and 2 patients had accelerated CLL. Three patients had non–CLL-related diagnoses (non–small cell lung cancer) metastatic neuroendocrine tumor and atypical pneumonia.[33] The investigators selected a cutoff point of SUV greater than or equal to 5 and found 91% sensitivity and 80% specificity for distinguishing RT from CLL, with a positive predictive value (PPV) of 53% and negative predictive value (NPV) of 97%.

Papajik and colleagues[35] performed a prospective study in 44 patients with newly diagnosed CLL, relapsed CLL, and RT. Twenty-three patients had PET/CT with newly diagnosed CLL with high disease burden, and 13 patients had PET/CT at the time of disease progression. PET/CT was positive (FDG avid) in 57% of patients with newly diagnosed CLL and was not avid in 43% of patients at the time of initial diagnosis. A higher percentage of PET/CTs were positive at the time of relapse (69%). Median SUV ranges were 3.4 and 3.1, respectively. Eight patients with RT had PET/CTs performed, 5 in the setting of suspicion for RT and 3 after histologic confirmation of RT. In patients with RT (suspected at the time of PET/CT or histologically confirmed), the median SUV_{max} was 16.5.[35] Five patients had RT (DLBCL) confirmed on biopsy of the most FDG-avid lymph node. PET/CT also identified 2 cases of HL and 1 case of anaplastic lymphoma kinase (ALK)-positive T-cell anaplastic large cell lymphoma. The investigators did not specify if the cases of HL were RT. Eight patients with bulky adenopathy (5 relapsed patients and 3 newly

Study	Cases of Richter Transformation	Maximum Standardized Uptake Value Cutoff	Sensitivity (%)	Specificity (%)	Positive Predictive Value (%)	Negative Predictive Value (%)
Bruzzi et al,[33] 2006	10	5	91	80	53	97
Mauro et al,[38] 2015	17	5	87	71.2	51.3	94
Falchi et al,[36] 2014	95	5	88	47	38	92
Michallet et al,[37] 2016	24	10	91	95	28.7	99.8
Mato et al,[39] 2017	8	10	71	50	26	88

Table 1
Summary of PET/CT predictive value for detecting Richter transformation

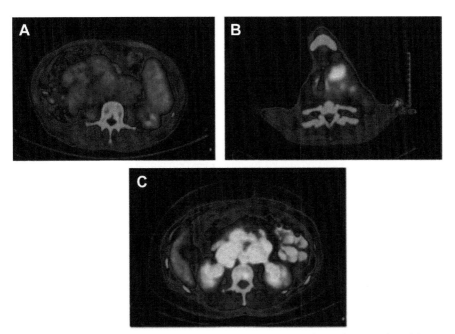

Fig. 1. Representative images of PET/CT imaging in patients with CLL, accelerated CLL, and RT. (*A*) PET/CT imaging of a patient with indolent CLL at diagnosis (SUV$_{max}$ 3). (*B*) PET/CT imaging of a patient with biopsy-proved accelerated CLL (SUV$_{max}$ 6). (*C*) PET/CT imaging of a patient with biopsy-proved RT (SUV$_{max}$ 29.4).

diagnosed patients) had histologically confirmed CLL. All patients with CLL had SUV$_{max}$ less than 7. The median OS for patients with RT was 8 months from diagnosis of RT and 36 months from initial diagnosis of CLL. This study demonstrated the utility of PET/CT to guide biopsy to diagnose RT and was the first to examine PET/CTs as a prognostic tool in CLL.

As a follow-up to the initial work performed by Bruzzi and colleagues, Falchi and colleagues[36] performed a single-center retrospective cohort to determine if PET/CT could predict RT and determine prognosis. They identified 764 CLL patients who underwent PET/CT for various indications, including concern for RT, initial staging, evaluation prior to or after treatment or prior to stem cell transplant, and staging for other malignancies; 332 patients had tissue biopsies, of which 95 (28.6%) were classified RT, 117 (35.2%) were classified as histologically aggressive CLL (HAC), and 120 (36.2%) were classified as histologically indolent (HIC) CLL. HAC was defined as CLL with increased large cells, large confluent proliferation centers, or high proliferation rate assessed by Ki-67. The median SUV$_{max}$ was 17.6 for patients with RT, 6.8 for patients with HAC, and 3.7 for patients with HIC; 88% of patients with RT had SUV$_{max}$ greater than or equal to 5 compared with 34% of patients with HIC.[36] The median survival was 7.7 months for patients with RT, 17.6 months for HAC, and not reached for HIC (*P*<.001). Using

an SUV$_{max}$ greater than or equal to 5, PET/CT had sensitivity of 91% and specificity 80% for RT, with PPV of 53% and NPV of 97%. Investigators also found that SUV$_{max}$ greater than or equal to 10 was associated with decreased OS for each histologic subtype compared with less than 10 (6 months vs 21 months for RT, *P* = .015; 7 mo vs 29 mo for HAC, *P* = .001; and 42 months vs not reached for HIC, *P* = .017, respectively). This study demonstrated an association between the intensity of FDG avidity with histologic subtype and demonstrated an association with increased FDG avidity (defined as SUV$_{max}$ ≥10) in both the CLL and RT histologic subtypes.

To further examine the utility of PET/CT in detecting RT, Michallet and colleagues[37] studied 240 patients (70 from Lyon Sud and Créteil Hospital Center and 170 from Mayo Clinic) with CLL who underwent PET/CT as part of clinical management. PET/CTs prior to treatment were performed and compared with post-treatment PET/CT if available. All patients had a biopsy within 1 month of their baseline scan. In this cohort, 10% of patients had RT, 42% had aggressive CLL (defined as histologic features of progression, including increased large cells, large confluent proliferation center, and high Ki-67 proliferation index), and 34% had stable disease (HIC CLL); 14% of patients underwent PET/CT for reasons unrelated to CLL.[37] The median tumor SUV$_{max}$ was 2.2 for patients with stable disease, 4.5 for aggressive

CLL, and 12.9 for RT. Differences between SUV_{max} for patients with RT versus stable CLL (12.9 vs 2.2; $P<.001$) and RT versus aggressive CLL (12.9 vs 4.5; $P<.001$) were statistically significant. An SUV_{max} cutoff of greater than or equal to 10 was effective in identifying RT (sensitivity 91% and specificity 95%) with NPV of 99% regardless of RT prevalence. The area under the curve for the receiver operating characteristic curve (ROC) for SUV_{max} greater than or equal to 10 was 95%. As in previous studies, PET/CT findings were correlated with OS (56.7 months SUV_{max} <10 vs 6.9 months $SUV_{max} \geq 10$). The investigators concluded an SUV_{max} of greater than or equal to 10 can distinguish RT in patients with CLL.

Mauro and colleagues[38] studied 90 CLL patients who underwent PET/CT imaging with subsequent biopsy if there was concern for RT or a secondary malignancy. The lymph node or tissue with the highest SUV_{max}, or if SUV_{max} less than 3 and overall distribution of SUV were similar, the largest palpable lymph node was biopsied. Eighty-nine PET/CTs were evaluated with median SUV_{max} of 4.5 (range 1.0–35.0); 84% of biopsies were of nodal sites and 16% were of extranodal sites. Biopsies revealed CLL/small lymphocytic lymphoma (SLL) in 74% of patients and RT in 19% (11% DLBCL and 8% HL), and 7% had a secondary malignancy. The median SUV_{max} for all patients with RT was 10 (3.5–36), 14.6 in patients with DLBCL, and 7 in HL. The median SUV_{max} was 3.5 in patients with tissue diagnosis of CLL/ SLL. Clinical and biological characteristics associated with SUV_{max} greater than or equal to 5 included presence of B symptoms, Binet stage B/C disease, bulky lymph nodes (≥ 5 cm), elevated ILDH and elevated β_2-microglobulin. A Ki-67 expression of greater than or equal to 30% was commonly seen when SUV_{max} greater than or equal to 5. IGHV mutation and 17p deletion were not associated with an SUV_{max} greater than or equal to 5. An SUV_{max} cutoff of greater than or equal to 5 demonstrated a sensitivity of 87% and, specificity of 71.2% for RT, with PPV of 51.3% and NPV of 94%. OS at 40 months was 13% for patients with DLBCL diagnosis, 83% for patients with HL, and 63% for patients with CLL/ SLL ($P = .0247$).

Recent data suggest worse outcomes for patients with RT previously treated with BCRis (including ibrutinib and idelalisib).[25,26] Mato and colleagues[39] performed a post hoc analysis of pretreatment PET/CTs from 167 patients enrolled in a phase 2, open-label, multicenter trial of patients treated venetoclax monotherapy after failing BCRi therapy; 50% of patients had a lymph node with SUV_{max} greater than or equal to 5 and 15%

had SUV_{max} greater than or equal to 10. Per protocol, 57 patients required pretreatment biopsies to rule out RT, 19 patients with SUV_{max} greater than or equal to 10 and 16 patients with SUV_{max} less than 10, with additional high-risk clinical/laboratory features concerning for RT; 22 patients failed screening for other reasons and did not have a biopsy. Eight of 57 patients who underwent biopsy had histologically confirmed RT (5 $SUV_{max} \geq 10$, 2 SUV_{max} <10, and 1 did not have a baseline PET). Fourteen patients with SUV_{max} greater than 10 had a biopsy that demonstrated CLL. Based on the results of Michallet and colleagues, a cutoff of SUV_{max} greater than or equal to 10 was used, and PET/CT in this study had a sensitivity of 71%, specificity of 50%, PPV of 26%, and NPV of 88% for detection of RT versus CLL (receiver operating characteristic area of 61%). There was no difference in sensitivity if the cutoff was lowered to SUV_{max} greater than or equal to 5 (71%), but specificity was decreased (4%) compared with SUV_{max} greater than or equal to 10; 127 patients subsequently were treated with venetoclax monotherapy and were evaluable for response. There were no differences in response rates to treatment with venetoclax when patients were stratified by SUV_{max} greater than or equal to 10 or SUV_{max} less than 10 (65% vs 62%, respectively), but the median PFS was longer for patients with SUV_{max} less than 10 (24.7 months; 95% CI, 20.1, not reached) versus SUV_{max} greater than or equal to 10 (15.4 months; 95% CI, 0.4, - $P = .033$)

SUMMARY

To date, several studies using PET/CT have demonstrated its value in evaluating patients with CLL for RT, with both high sensitivity and high specificity. In patients treated with BCRi, PET/CT has lower sensitivity and specificity compared with earlier studies in patients treated with CIT, possibly due to treatment effects with these agents on cellular metabolic function. The NPV remains excellent and SUV_{max} of greater than or equal to 10 remains an important tool for detecting RT in patients treated with either CIT or BCRi. Although PET/CT is useful in detecting RT, the results should be used to guide the need for and choice of biopsy site and cannot replace a tissue diagnosis. SUV_{max} for patients with HL and DLBCL differed across studies, with HL having a lower SUV_{max}. Studies of HL RT are ongoing.[40] Higher SUV_{max} was associated with shorter PFS in patients with CLL and RT, although further prospective studies are needed to determine its role in prognostication, particularly in the era of chemotherapy-free regimens. Based on current data, if RT is suspected, PET/CT can be used to identify a site for biopsy to confirm clinical suspicion. For patients treated with novel agents, the test characteristics for PET indicate that it is somewhat less helpful in this regard (modestly diminished sensitivity and specificity). Whether PET/CT should be used to prognosticate patients receiving therapy for CLL remains an area of debate, particularly because risk-adaptive approaches have not been tested based on pretreatment PET CT results.

REFERENCES

1. Noone A, Howlader N, Krapcho M, et al. SEER cancer statistics review, 1975-2015. Bethesda (MD): National Cancer Institute; 2017. Accessed November 15, 2018.
2. Hallek M, Cheson BD, Catovsky D, et al. iwCLL guidelines for diagnosis, indications for treatment, response assessment, and supportive management of CLL. Blood 2018;131(25):2745–60.
3. Hallek M, Cheson BD, Catovsky D, et al. Guidelines for the diagnosis and treatment of chronic lymphocytic leukemia: a report from the International Workshop on Chronic Lymphocytic Leukemia updating the National Cancer Institute-Working Group 1996 guidelines. Blood 2008;111(12):5446–56.
4. Rai KR, Sawitsky A, Cronkite EP, et al. Clinical staging of chronic lymphocytic leukemia. Blood 1975; 46(2):219–34.
5. Binet JL, Leporrier M, Dighiero G, et al. A clinical staging system for chronic lymphocytic leukemia: prognostic significance. Cancer 1977;40(2):855–64.
6. International CLL-IPI working group. An international prognostic index for patients with chronic lymphocytic leukaemia (CLL-IPI): a meta-analysis of individual patient data. Lancet Oncol 2016;17(6):779–90.
7. Döhner H, Stilgenbauer S, Benner A, et al. Genomic aberrations and survival in chronic lymphocytic leukemia. N Engl J Med 2000;343(26):1910–6.
8. Gonzalez D, Martinez P, Wade R, et al. Mutational status of the TP53 gene as a predictor of response and survival in patients with chronic lymphocytic leukemia: results from the LRF CLL4 trial. J Clin Oncol 2011;29(16):2223–9.
9. Tam CS, Shanafelt TD, Wierda WG, et al. De novo deletion 17p13.1 chronic lymphocytic leukemia shows significant clinical heterogeneity: the M. D. Anderson and Mayo Clinic experience. Blood 2009;114(5):957–64.
10. Damle RN, Wasil T, Fais F, et al. Ig V Gene Mutation Status and CD38 Expression As Novel Prognostic Indicators in Chronic Lymphocytic Leukemia. Presented in part at the 40th Annual Meeting of The American Society of Hematology, held in Miami Beach, FL, December 4–8, 1998. 1999;94(6):1840-1847.
11. Hamblin TJ, Davis Z, Gardiner A, et al. Unmutated Ig V_H genes are associated with a more aggressive form of chronic lymphocytic leukemia. Blood 1999; 94(6):1848–54.
12. Hallek M, Fischer K, Fingerle-Rowson G, et al. Addition of rituximab to fludarabine and cyclophosphamide in patients with chronic lymphocytic leukaemia: a randomised, open-label, phase 3 trial. Lancet 2010; 376(9747):1164–74.
13. Fischer K, Bahlo J, Fink A-M, et al. Extended follow up of the CLL8 protocol, a randomized phase-III trial of the German CLL Study Group (GCLLSG) comparing fludarabine and cyclophosphamide (FC) to FC plus rituximab (FCR) for previously untreated patients with chronic lymphocytic leukemia (CLL): results on survival, progression-free survival, delayed Neutropenias and secondary malignancies confirm superiority of the FCR regimen. Blood 2012; 120(21):435.
14. Fischer K, Cramer P, Busch R, et al. Bendamustine in combination with rituximab for previously untreated patients with chronic lymphocytic leukemia: a multicenter phase II trial of the German Chronic Lymphocytic Leukemia Study Group. J Clin Oncol 2012;30(26):3209–16.
15. Quinquenel A, Willekens C, Dupuis J, et al. Bendamustine and rituximab combination in the management of chronic lymphocytic leukemia-associated autoimmune hemolytic anemia: a multicentric retrospective study of the French CLL intergroup (GCFLLC/MW and GOELAMS). Am J Hematol 2015;90(3):204–7.
16. Tsimberidou AM, O'Brien S, Khouri I, et al. Clinical outcomes and prognostic factors in patients with Richter's syndrome treated with chemotherapy or chemoimmunotherapy with or without stem-cell transplantation. J Clin Oncol 2006;24(15):2343–51.
17. Rossi D, Spina V, Deambrogi C, et al. The genetics of Richter syndrome reveals disease heterogeneity and predicts survival after transformation. Blood 2011;117(12):3391–401.
18. Parikh SA, Rabe KG, Call TG, et al. Diffuse large B-cell lymphoma (Richter syndrome) in patients with chronic lymphocytic leukaemia (CLL): a cohort study of newly diagnosed patients. Br J Haematol 2013;162(6):774–82.
19. Jenke P, Eichhorst B, Busch R, et al. Cyclophosphamide, adriamycin, vincristine and prednisone plus rituximab (CHOP-R) in fludarabine (F) refractory chronic lymphocytic leukemia (CLL) or CLL with autoimmune cytopenia (AIC) or Richter's transformation (RT): final analysis of a phase II study of the German CLL Study Group 2011;118(21):2860.
20. Tsimberidou AM, Kantarjian HM, Cortes J, et al. Fractionated cyclophosphamide, vincristine, liposomal

daunorubicin, and dexamethasone plus rituximab and granulocyte-macrophage-colony stimulating factor (GM-CSF) alternating with methotrexate and cytarabine plus rituximab and GM-CSF in patients with Richter syndrome or fludarabine-refractory chronic lymphocytic leukemia. Cancer 2003;97(7):1711–20.

21. Dabaja BS, O'Brien SM, Kantarjian HM, et al. Fractionated cyclophosphamide, vincristine, liposomal daunorubicin (daunoXome), and dexamethasone (hyperCVXD) regimen in Richter's syndrome. Leuk Lymphoma 2001;42(3):329–37.

22. Rossi D, Gaidano G. Richter syndrome: pathogenesis and management. Semin Oncol 2016;43(2): 311–9.

23. Mato AR, Nabhan C, Barr PM, et al. Outcomes of CLL patients treated with sequential kinase inhibitor therapy: a real world experience. Blood 2016; 128(18):2199–205.

24. Ayers EC, Mato AR. Richter's transformation in the era of kinase inhibitor therapy: a review. Clin Lymphoma Myeloma Leuk 2017;17(1):1–6.

25. Jain P, Keating M, Wierda W, et al. Outcomes of patients with chronic lymphocytic leukemia after discontinuing ibrutinib. Blood 2015;125(13):2062–7.

26. Maddocks KJ, Ruppert AS, Lozanski G, et al. Etiology of ibrutinib therapy discontinuation and outcomes in patients with chronic lymphocytic leukemia. JAMA Oncol 2015;1(1):80–7.

27. Tsimberidou AM, Wierda WG, Plunkett W, et al. Phase I-II study of oxaliplatin, fludarabine, cytarabine, and rituximab combination therapy in patients with Richter's syndrome or fludarabine-refractory chronic lymphocytic leukemia. J Clin Oncol 2008; 26(2):196–203.

28. Chigrinova E, Rinaldi A, Kwee I, et al. Two main genetic pathways lead to the transformation of chronic lymphocytic leukemia to Richter syndrome. Blood 2013;122(15):2673–82.

29. Rossi D, Rasi S, Fabbri G, et al. Mutations of NOTCH1 are an independent predictor of survival in chronic lymphocytic leukemia. Blood 2012; 119(2):521–9.

30. Rossi D, Rasi S, Spina V, et al. Different impact of NOTCH1 and SF3B1 mutations on the risk of chronic lymphocytic leukemia transformation to Richter syndrome. Br J Haematol 2012;158(3):426–9.

31. Rossi D, Spina V, Cerri M, et al. Stereotyped B-cell receptor is an independent risk factor of chronic lymphocytic leukemia transformation to Richter syndrome. Clin Cancer Res 2009;15(13):4415–22.

32. Mayr C, Speicher MR, Kofler DM, et al. Chromosomal translocations are associated with poor prognosis in chronic lymphocytic leukemia. Blood 2006; 107(2):742–51.

33. Bruzzi JF, Macapinlac H, Tsimberidou AM, et al. Detection of Richter's transformation of chronic lymphocytic leukemia by PET/CT. J Nucl Med 2006; 47(8):1267–73.

34. Karam M, Novak L, Cyriac J, et al. Role of fluorine-18 fluoro-deoxyglucose positron emission tomography scan in the evaluation and follow-up of patients with low-grade lymphomas. Cancer 2006;107(1): 175–83.

35. Papajik T, Myslivecek M, Urbanova R, et al. 2-[18F] fluoro-2-deoxy-D-glucose positron emission tomography/computed tomography examination in patients with chronic lymphocytic leukemia may reveal Richter transformation. Leuk Lymphoma 2014;55(2):314–9.

36. Falchi L, Keating MJ, Marom EM, et al. Correlation between FDG/PET, histology, characteristics, and survival in 332 patients with chronic lymphoid leukemia. Blood 2014;123(18):2783–90.

37. Michallet AS, Sesques P, Rabe KG, et al. An 18F-FDG-PET maximum standardized uptake value > 10 represents a novel valid marker for discerning Richter's Syndrome. Leuk Lymphoma 2016;57(6):1474–7.

38. Mauro FR, Chauvie S, Paoloni F, et al. Diagnostic and prognostic role of PET/CT in patients with chronic lymphocytic leukemia and progressive disease. Leukemia 2015;29(6):1360–5.

39. Mato AR, Wierda WG, Davids MS, et al. Analysis of PET-CT to identify Richter's transformation in 167 patients with disease progression following kinase inhibitor therapy. Blood 2017;130(Suppl 1):834.

40. Stephens DM, Boucher K, Kander E, et al. Chronic lymphocytic leukemia (CLL) transformed into Hodgkin lymphoma (HL): clinical characteristics and outcomes from a large multi-center Collaboration 2018; 132(Suppl 1):1648.

PET-Computed Tomography in Myeloma

Current Overview and Future Directions

Deepu Madduri, MD*, Bart Barlogie, MD

KEYWORDS

• Multiple myeloma • PET/CT • IMWG criteria • Smoldering myeloma • Solitary plasmacytoma

KEY POINTS

- The treatment landscape of multiple myeloma has been rapidly evolving and International Myeloma Working Group has published modified diagnostic criteria.
- Whole body skeletal survey has been considered "gold standard," now PET/computed tomography (CT) more widely used.
- PET/CT can help predict risk progression from smoldering myeloma and identify patients with solitary plasmacytoma.
- PET/CT helps learn the extent of bone marrow involvement in patients with active myeloma.
- PET/CT helps identify extramedullary disease.

BACKGROUND

Multiple myeloma (MM) is a malignancy involving plasma cells. It includes a spectrum of plasma cell disorders ranging from monoclonal gammopathy of unknown significance, a relatively benign condition, to smoldering MM and the symptomatic malignant disorder MM and its more aggressive form, plasma cell leukemia with circulating myeloma cells in the blood as well as extramedullary disease. MM is characterized by the presence of clonal plasma cells that secrete monoclonal immunoglobulins in most cases and lead to organ dysfunction. Generally, the clonal plasma cells can produce any 1 of the 5 immunoglobulin subtypes, mainly immunoglobulin G (IgG) and IgA. In about 30%, heavy-chain components of the immunoglobulin molecule are not secreted, referred to light-chain MM (kappa [κ] or lambda [λ] type). Another 10% are nonsecretory MM, a condition that frequently emerges as the end stage of MM.

One characteristic of MM is the presence of osteolytic bone lesions that can cause hypercalcemia, severe bone pain, pathologic fractures, and spinal cord compression. The bone destruction is a major cause of morbidity and mortality.[1] At diagnosis, up to 10% of the patients may have osteopenia or osteoporosis.[2] The use of steroids for myeloma treatment can also exacerbate osteopenia and osteoporosis. Up to 90% of patients with myeloma develop osteolytic lesions during the course of their disease.[3] The axial skeleton, particularly the spine, is the most often affected. Other bones such as ribs (45%), skull and shoulders (40%), sternum and pelvis (30%), and long bones (25%) are also affected.[4,5] Osteolysis results from increased osteoclastic activity and impaired osteoblastogenesis, which accounts for persistence of lytic lesions even in patients responding to treatment.[2,6–10] Impairment of osteoblast function explains radioisotope bone scans are typically negative in patients with lytic lesions.[11] Appropriate use of imaging techniques is essential in the identification and characterization of the skeletal complications resulting from MM and in determining the extent of intramedullary

Disclosure Statement: The authors have nothing to disclose.
Mount Sinai Hospital/Tisch Cancer Institute, 1 Gustave L Levy Place, Box 1185, New York, NY 10029, USA
* Corresponding author.
E-mail address: Deepu.Madduri@mountsinai.org

PET Clin 14 (2019) 411–418
https://doi.org/10.1016/j.cpet.2019.03.010
1556-8598/19/

and extramedullary disease.[1] It is clear despite knowing the importance of imaging patients with newly diagnosed MM, and for patients who we are following through a course of treatment, that we as a group often lack a standardized imaging approach. International Myeloma Working Group (IMWG) has created consensus criteria for disease response but imaging criteria have not yet widely been adopted.[10,12]

Lytic lesions are generally diagnosed by radiographic analysis, which is considered as a gold standard of the imaging modalities in MM. The presence of bone lesions generally require treatment even in the absence of clinical symptoms and end organ damage (CRAB; hypercalcemia, renal insufficiency, anemia, and bone disease).[13] Since 1903, when Weber first observed that myeloma lesions are evident on radiographs, X rays have been extensively used to identify myeloma-related bone lesions both at diagnosis and during disease course.[1] In flat bones of the skull and pelvis, lytic lesions look like punched-out lesions without reactive sclerosis of the surrounding bone.[14] Lytic lesions, in the long bones, can appear as mottled areas of multiple small lesions or have endosteal scalloping.[15] Even with complete radiographic X rays, almost 10% to 20% of lytic lesions are missed. Bone X rays are also not specific so that benign causes of osteopenia are confused with lytic lesions.[16] Some bones on the X rays are not well visualized and one may need multiple views of a bone to get an accurate diagnosis. One other issue with X rays is that it fails to show response to treatment as these lesions rarely heal with response to therapy.[8] For all these reasons, although conventional X rays are considered as a "gold standard" for the determination of the extent of myeloma bone disease at diagnosis, computed tomography (CT) or MR imaging have been used to increase the sensitivity and specificity of early detection of myeloma-associated bone destruction. Using these modalities, it is possible to visualize soft tissue involvement and/or distinguish between malignant and benign compression fractures. In recent years, PET has also been used in MM imaging.

Over the past decade, the treatment landscape for MM has been rapidly changing with the addition of several new classes of drugs with varying mechanisms of action.[17–19] The landscape is further changing over the past 2 years with the introduction of bispecific antibodies (bispecific T-cell engager) and chimeric antigen receptor cell therapy leading to improved survival for patients with MM.[20,21] Given the plethora of effective treatment strategies, it is important to have not only better response criteria but also better

imaging tools to measure treatment response. The IMWG has considerably evolved the response criteria and clarified that more than one focal lesion on MR imaging and one or more lytic bone lesions detected on CT scan, including whole-body low-dose CT or PET/CT, fulfill the criteria for bone damage requiring therapy.[10,22] The IMWG also make recommendations for serial imaging in patients with extramedullary disease and/or solitary plasmacytoma.[10,22] This article focuses mostly on the imaging modalities used in myeloma, focusing primarily on PET/CT uses in the myeloma world.

PET-COMPUTED TOMOGRAPHY IMAGING SCANS

PET is a tomographic nuclear imaging procedure that uses positrons as radiolabels and positron-electron annihilation reaction γ-rays to locate the radiolabels. A low dose of a radiopharmaceutical labeled with a positron emitter, such as 18-fluorine-fluorodeoxyglucose (FDG), is injected into the patient, who is scanned by a tomographic system.[1] Given the poor spatial resolution of the PET scan, it is often combined with CT.[23] Tumor cells have increased metabolism, which can be detected on PET/CT. The sensitivity of FDG-PET in detecting myelomatous involvement is approximately 85% and its specificity is 92%.[23] In general, PET/CT is reliable in recognizing lesions at least 1 cm or above, and a standard standardized uptake value (SUV) cutoff of 2.5 is used to identify presence of disease.[24] If the lesions are less than 5 mm in diameter, it is recommended any amount of FDG uptake should be considered positive, regardless of SUV. If the SUV is less than 2.5 and the lesions are between 5 and 10 mm, then it is considered intermediate. Reading PET scans are operator dependent. In addition, the patient's body mass and weight affect SUV as well.[23,24] One of the pivotal studies in 2002 assessed 66 patients who were observed serially and determined that PET/CT can be used to identify patients with high-risk myeloma and monitor nonsecretory myeloma.[25] This study helped put MM on the map as a disease that should be incorporated into larger studies of PET/CT in the United States.[26,27] Here is an image of a patient who had nonsecretory myeloma, which is difficult to follow with serum blood immunoglobulins, followed by PET/CT imaging before and after chemotherapy (**Fig. 1**).[28] After the National Oncologic PET Registry showed that 36.5% of the physicians changed their intended management based on PET/CT results, the NCCN guidelines added PET/CT as a tool to diagnose and monitor myeloma.[26]

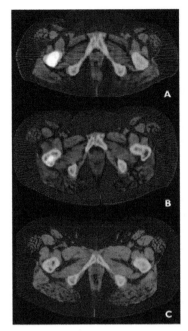

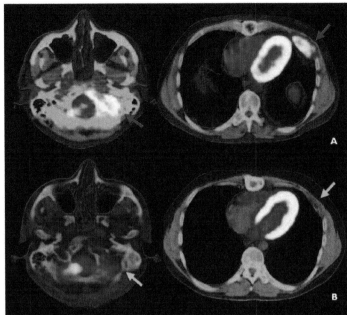

Fig. 1. Complete metabolic response after chemotherapy in a 44-year-old patient with nonsecretory plasmacytomas presenting with recurrent disease and restarted on systemic chemotherapy. (*A*) Pretreatment axial fused PET/CT image shows ^{18}F-FDG-avid plasmacytomas involving left clivus (maximum SUV, 5.8) and left anterior fifth rib (*red arrows*) with no evidence of other bone lesion. (*B*) Posttherapy (6 months after restart of chemotherapy) axial fused PET/CT image shows complete metabolic resolution in left skull base and left fifth rib plasmacytomas (*blue arrows*), consistent with excellent therapy response. Patient remained free of disease in 5-year follow-up.

Currently, the most widely used PET tracer for MM is ^{18}F-FDG. There are multiple new PET/CT tracers that are being studied in a limited series of patients.[29] The tracers target different metabolic pathways or receptors expressed on plasma cells and act as molecular imaging biomarkers. The limited sizes in these varying studies do not support the superiority of any of these tracers over the standard ^{18}F-FDG tracer. Additional studies should be done to help us understand the proper tracer to use while assessing patient's response to therapy.

In newly diagnosed MM, a prospective study comparing 3 different imaging modalities (PET/CT, MR imaging, and whole-body X rays) showed that the PET/CT was superior to plain X rays in 46% of the patients, including 19% with negative X rays (**Table 1**); 35% of the patients had myelomatous lesions detected on a PET/CT that were out of the field view of an MR imaging. On the contrary, PET/CT did not show any abnormal bone findings in 30% of the patients who had diffuse bone marrow involvement on MR imaging. Therefore, combining both PET/CT and MR imaging allows the detection of both medullary and extramedullary MM.[30] Whole body X rays are found to have a higher sensitivity to depict lesions in the skull and ribs. Other false positives with a

PET/CT might occur with the presence of bone metallic implants and accumulation of tracer into physiologically active sites such as kidneys, bladder, and ureters. Use of growth factors can induce a false diffuse marrow pattern. Another big limitation is hyperglycemia or recent administration of high dose of steroids, which can lead to transient metabolic suppression.[31,32] Furthermore, a small subset of patients with MM may not express glucose transporter (GLUT-1) or the plasma cells may not be FDG avid, therefore making it very difficult to distinguish between a low metabolic lesion related to MM and a benign one.[30,33]

SMOLDERING MYELOMA

Smoldering myeloma is defined by the IMWG criteria as serum M-protein less than 3 g/dL and/or less than 10% monoclonal plasma cells in the bone marrow in the absence of myeloma-defining events, including absence of focal lesions on imaging (**Box 1**).[22,34] The role of ^{18}F-FDG PET/CT in predicting the risk of progression of smoldering MM to active MM is very limited. In one study, the risk of progression to active MM was about 75% in patients with smoldering myeloma with increased ^{18}F-FDG uptake despite not

Table 1
Imaging limitations by modality

Imaging Modality	Limitations
Conventional radiology	• Some areas not well visualized • Limited sensitivity (10%–20%) of lesions are missed • Reduced specificity vs benign causes of osteopenia (steroids, postmenopausal) • Fail to show response to treatment • Observer dependent
PET/CT	• Lack of standardization • High costs • Observer dependent • Not available at all institutions/hospitals • Suboptimal in detecting diffuse bone marrow plasma cell infiltration and lytic lesions in skull • False positivity due to bone metallic implants, tracer in physiologic active sites • False positivity due to hyperglycemia or recent use of high-dose steroids
MR imaging	• Patient intolerance due to duration of study • Cardiac pacemakers • Intraorbital foreign bodies • Limited field area to visualize lesions • False diffuse marrow pattern due to G-CSF use

Abbreviation: G-CSF, granulocyte-colony stimulating factor.

exhibiting underlying lytic lesions.[35] Another prospective study suggests that focal lesions without underlying bone changes on ^{18}F-FDG PET/CT scans predict for a higher risk of early progression from smoldering myeloma to active MM.[36] In this study, the 19 of 120 patients who had a positive ^{18}F-FDG PET/CT scan had a 58% risk of progression to active MM and shorter time to progression (median 1.1 years). The patients with negative ^{18}F-FDG PET/CT scans had a 33% risk of progression at 2 years and median time to progression was 4.5 years.[36] Therefore, patients who meet the criteria for smoldering myeloma but have one or more lytic lesions on [118]F-FDG PET/CT scans should be defined as having active MM and be

initiated on therapy. If skeletal survey is negative and whole-body MR imaging is unavailable, IMWG recommends PET/CT to distinguish active MM from smoldering myeloma.[29]

SOLITARY PLASMACYTOMA

Solitary plasmacytoma is an infiltration of abnormal plasma cells that grow within the soft tissue or bony skeleton. The diagnosis of a solitary plasmacytoma relies on the biopsy showing presence of clonal plasma cells, either in the absence of bone marrow plasma cell infiltration or with less than 10% plasma cells in the bone marrow and with no evidence of end organ damage. It is imperative to use imaging modalities to rule out other coexisting occult sites of disease because this affects the prognosis and treatment course. MR imaging of the axial skeletal has been shown to be superior than skeletal survey and recommended if patient has a solitary plasmacytoma of the spine.[37,38] This will help rule out any suspected cord compression. In a meta-analysis of 14 studies, ^{18}F-FDG PET/CT was regarded as having the highest reliability in terms of sensitivity and specificity for detection of clonal plasma cells outside of the bone marrow.[39] IMWG, based on limited availability of whole-body MR imaging, recommend ^{18}F-FDG PET/CT as part of the initial investigations in patients with a suspicion of either extramedullary plasmacytoma or solitary bone plasmacytoma.[29]

ACTIVE MULTIPLE MYELOMA

Active MM is defined by the updated IMWG criteria as having greater than or equal to 60% plasma cells, greater than or equal to 100 involved/uninvolved serum free light-chain ratio, presence of lytic lesions, and/or having end organ damage.[34] ^{18}F-FDG PET/CT can be used to determine the prognosis of patients with newly diagnosed and relapsed or refractory myeloma. The presence of 3 or more lesions at baseline PET/CT scan, an independent factor, was linked to shortened progression-free survival and overall survival in patients who had upfront novel therapy and tandem autologous stem-cell transplants.[33] The same group published an updated data analysis and suggested that greater than 3 lesions on PET/CT and greater than 7 lesions on axial MR imaging was not only associated with a high-risk gene expression profile (GEP) score but also seen in patients with extramedullary disease.[40] Another study done by the same group evaluated prognostic implications of 3 imaging tools (skeletal survey, MR imaging, and PET/CT) in 2 consecutive Total Therapy 3 trials

---

Box 1
Definition of multiple myeloma based on 2014 IMWG criteria

Panel: Revised International Myeloma Working Group diagnostic criteria for multiple myeloma and smouldering multiple myeloma

Definition of multiple myeloma

Clonal bone marrow plasma cells ≥10% or biopsy-proven bony or extramedullary plasmacytoma[a] and any one or more of the following myeloma-defining events:

- Myeloma-defining events:
  - Evidence of end-organ damage that can be attributed to the underlying plasma cell proliferative disorder, specifically:
    - Hypercalcaemia: serum calcium >0.25 mmol/L (>1 mg/dL) higher than the upper limit of normal or >2.75 mmol/L (>11 mg/dL)
    - Renal insufficiency: creatinine clearance less than 40 mL/min[b] or serum creatinine >177 μmol/L (>2 mg/dL)
    - Anemia: hemoglobin value of >20 g/L less than the lower limit of normal or a hemoglobin value <100 g/L
    - Bone lesions: one or more osteolytic lesions on skeletal radiography, CT, or PET-CT[c]
  - Any one or more of the following biomarkers of malignancy:
    - Clonal bone marrow plasma cell percentage[a] ≥60%
    - Involved:uninvolved serum free light-chain ratio[d] ≥100
    - >1 focal lesions on MR imaging studies[e]

Definition of smouldering multiple myeloma

Both criteria must be met:

- Serum monoclonal protein (IgG or IgA) ≥30 g/L or urinary monoclonal protein ≥500 mg per 24 hours and/or clonal bone marrow plasma cells 10% to 60%
- Absence of myeloma-defining events or amyloidosis

PET-CT-^{18}F-FDG PET with CT.

[a] Clonality should be established by showing κ/λ light-chain restriction on flow cytometry, immunohistochemistry, or immunofluorescence. Bone marrow plasma cell percentage should preferably be estimated from a core biopsy specimen; in case of a disparity between the aspirate and core biopsy, the highest value should be used.
[b] Measured or estimated by validated equations.
[c] If bone marrow has less than 10% clonal plasma cells, more than one bone lesion is required to distinguish from solitary plasmacytoma with minimal marrow involvement.
[d] These values are based on the serum Freelite assay (The Binding Site Group, Birmingham, UK). The involved free light chain must be greater than or equal to 100 mg/L.
[e] Each focal lesion must be 5 mm or more in size.
Both criteria must be fulfilled.
From Rajkumar SV, Dimopoulos MA, Palumbo A, et al. International Myeloma Working Group updated criteria for the diagnosis of multiple myeloma. Lancet Oncol 2014;15:e538–48; with permission.

---

for newly diagnosed patients with myeloma. A PET/CT was done at baseline and on day 7 of induction as well as GEP testing. According to their multivariate analysis, the presence of more than 3 focal lesions on day 7 with GEP high-risk disease showed inferior overall survival and progression-free survival.[41] In addition, complete suppression of FDG avidity in focal lesions before an autologous transplant was associated with longer progression-free survival and overall survival.

In patients with relapsed disease after an autologous transplant or allogeneic transplant, a negative PET/CT scan confirmed favorable prognosis.[42] However, greater than 10 lesions on PET/CT scan especially in the appendicular skeleton and the presence of extramedullary disease adversely affected both time to progression and overall survival. SUV value greater than 18.6 is also associated with shorter time to progression. Another study highlights the value of PET/CT in detecting sites of active disease at the time of relapse or progression with a 100% specificity and 80% sensitivity.[43] When all these data are combined, it is clear that evaluation of metabolic

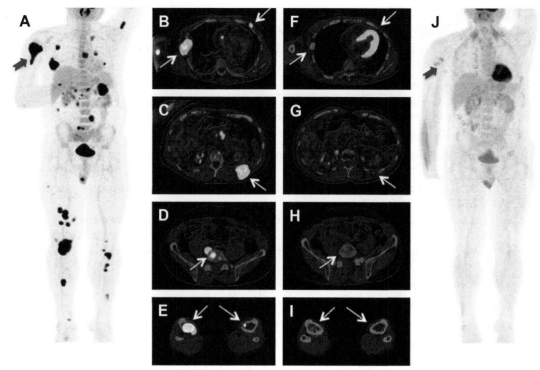

Fig. 2. Whole-body ^{18}FDG-PET/CT of a 48-year-old woman affected with MM and pathologic fracture of the right humerus, before and after chemotherapy and autologous stem cell transplantation. Pre- and posttherapy images: maximum intensity projection PET (*A, J*); axial PET/CT fused images of the chest (*B, F*), abdomen (*C, G*), pelvis (*D, H*), and lower limbs (*E, I*). Multiple skeletal lesions in the whole bone compartment both axial and appendicular (*A*) with extension to the surrounding soft tissues (*B–D*) were observed in the pretherapy examination. The posttherapy evaluation (*F–I*) showed good response to therapy with radiopharmaceutical uptake only in the right humerus (*J*), corresponding to the previous pathologic fracture (*red arrow*).

activity seen on ^{18}F-FDG PET/CT predict for earlier detection of relapse, confirm relapse or progression of disease, and in turn is a very useful tool in the prognostic identification of patients with myeloma.

Just as ^{18}F-FDG PET/CT is a helpful tool in determining prognosis, it is also an excellent tool in identifying response to treatment in patients with MM, because it can recognize metabolically active and inactive lesions. In a series of patients who were randomized to receive upfront autologous transplant or standard dose intensification therapy followed by 1 year of maintenance therapy, results showed that negative PET/CT scan after induction therapy had improved progression-free survival when compared with persistent PET/CT uptake.[44] Moreover, negative PET/CT before starting maintenance therapy also predicts for longer progression-free survival and overall survival. Various other studies also confirmed similar findings.[41,45] PET/CT is also associated with faster normalization of imaging findings than MR imaging.[46] In conclusion, IMWG recommends

that PET/CT scan should be the preferred imaging modality to monitor patient's response to therapy (**Fig. 2**).[47] In addition, PET/CT can also be coupled with minimal residual disease evaluation to detect presence of extramedullary disease.

SUMMARY

The improved treatment landscape of MM has contributed to improved survival for patients with MM. Given the effective treatment strategies, it is important to not only have better response criteria but also have effective imaging modalities to measure treatment response. Various imaging technologies have been used for the diagnosis and management of patients with myeloma. Whole-body skeletal survey has been considered as a "gold standard" for the determination of the extent of myeloma bone disease at diagnosis. However, MR imaging and PET/CT have been used to increase the sensitivity and specificity of early detection of myeloma-associated bone destruction. IMWG has published modified diagnostic criteria as well as imaging modality recommendations in patients with smoldering myeloma, solitary plasmacytomas, and active MM. PET/CT scans can also help predict for earlier detection of relapse, confirm relapse or progression of disease, and help with prognostic evaluation as well as monitor patient's response to therapy. In summary, although all reported studies have confirmed the superiority of PET/CT over conventional radiography, they have also revealed that if PET/CT was the sole imaging study done, it would miss many additional small lytic skeletal lesions and could miss diffuse spine involvement compared with MR imaging. Further targeted studies in myeloma are required to further clarify aspects of the specific utility of these imaging modalities in patients with myeloma. At this time, PET/CT is still recommended in patients with active myeloma, smoldering myeloma, and solitary plasmacytoma.

REFERENCES

1. Dimopoulos M, Terpos E, Comenzo RL, et al. International myeloma working group consensus statement and guidelines regarding the current role of imaging techniques in the diagnosis and monitoring of multiple myeloma. Leukemia 2009;23:1545–56.
2. Callander NS, Roodman GD. Myeloma bone disease. Semin Hematol 2001;38:276–85.
3. Kyle RA, Gertz MA, Witzig TE, et al. Review of 1027 patients with newly diagnosed multiple myeloma. Mayo Clin Proc 2003;78:21–33.
4. Terpos E, Dimopoulos MA. Myeloma bone disease: pathophysiology and management. Ann Oncol 2005;16:1223–31.
5. Healy CF, Murray JG, Eustace SJ, et al. Multiple myeloma: a review of imaging features and radiolocial techniques. Bone Marrow Res 2011;2011:439–583.
6. Epstein J, Walker R. Myeloma and bone disease: "the dangerous tango". Clin Adv Hematol Oncol 2006;4:300–6.
7. Giuliani N, Rizzoli V, Roodman GD. Multiple myeloma bone disease: pathophysiology of osteoblast inhibition. Blood 2006;108:3992–6.
8. Terpos E, Sezer O, Croucher P, et al. Myeloma bone disease and proteasome inhibition therapies. Blood 2007;110:1098–104.
9. Wahlin A, Holm J, Osterman G, et al. Evaluation of serial bone X-ray examination in multiple myeloma. Acta Med Scand 1982;212:385–7.
10. Kumar S, Paiva B, Anderson K, et al. International Myeloma Working group consensus criteria for response and minimal residual disease assessment in multiple myeloma. Lancet 2016;17:328–43.
11. Mileshkin L, Blum R, Seymour JF, et al. A comparison of fluorine-18 fluoro-deoxyglucose PET and technetium-99m sestamibi in assessing patients with multiple myeloma. Eur J Haematol 2004;72:32–7.
12. Mulligan ME, Badros AZ. PET/CT and MR imaging in myeloma. Skeletal Radiol 2007;36:5–16.
13. International Myeloma Working Group. Criteria for the classification of monoclonal gammopathies, multiple myeloma and related disorders: a report of the International Myeloma Working Group. Br J Haematol 2003;121:749–57.
14. Boccadoro M, Pileri A. Plasma cell dyscrasias: classification, clinical and laboratory characteristics, and differential diagnosis. Baillieres Clin Haematol 1995;8:705–19.
15. Agren B, Lönnqvist B, Björkstrand B, et al. Radiography and bone scintigraphy in bone marrow transplant multiple myeloma patients. Acta Radiol 1997;38:144–50.
16. Collins CD. Multiple myeloma. Cancer Imaging 2004;4(Spec No A):S47–53.
17. Kumar SK, Dispenzieri A, Lacy MQ, et al. Continued improvement in survival in multiple myeloma: changes in early mortality and outcomes in older patients. Leukemia 2013;28:1122–8.
18. Pozzi S, Marcheselli L, Bari A, et al. Survival of multiple myeloma patients in the era of novel therapies confirms the improvement in patients younger than 75 years: a population-based analysis. Br J Haematol 2013;163:40–6.
19. Rajkumar SV. IV. Initial treatment of multiple myeloma. Hematol Oncol 2013;31(suppl 1):33–7.
20. Raje NS, et al. bb2121 anti-BCMA CAR T-cell therapy in patients with relapsed/refractory multiple myeloma: updated results from a multicenter phase 1 study. 2018 ASCO Annual Meeting. Abstract 8007. Presented June 1, 2018.
21. Topp MS, Duell J, Zugmaier G, et al. Treatment with AMG 420, an Anti-B-Cell maturation antigen (BCMA) Bispecific T-cell engager (BiTE) antibody construct, induces minimal residual disease (MRD) negative complete responses in relapsed and/or refractory multiple myeloma patients: results of a first-in-human phase 1 dose escalation study. Blood 2018;132(suppl 1):1010.
22. Rajkumar SV, Dimopoulos MA, Palumbo A, et al. International Myeloma Working Group updated criteria for the diagnosis of multiple myeloma. Lancet Oncol 2014;15:e538–48.
23. Bredella MA, Steinbach L, Caputo G, et al. Value of FDG PET in the assessment of patients with multiple myeloma. AJR Am J Roentgenol 2005;184:1199–204.
24. Larson SM, Erdi Y, Akhurst T, et al. Tumor treatment response based on visual and quantitative changes in global tumor glycolysis using PET/FDG imaging. The visual response score and the change in total

lesion glycolysis. Clin Positron Imaging 1999;2: 159–71.

25. Durie BGM, Waxman AD, D'Agnolo A, et al. Whole-body F-FDG PET identifies high-risk myeloma. J Nucl Med 2002;43:1457–63.

26. Hillner BE, Siegel BA, Liu D, et al. Impact of positron emission tomography/computed tomography and positron emission tomography (PET) alone on expected management of patients with cancer: initial results from the National Oncologic PET Registry. J Clin Oncol 2008;26:2155–61.

27. Larson SM. Practice-based evidence of the beneficial impact of positron emission tomography in clinical oncology. J Clin Oncol 2008;26:2083–4.

28. Agarwal A, Chirindel A, Shah B, et al. Evolving role of FDG PET/CT in multiple myeloma imaging and management. Am J Roentgenol 2013;200(4):884–90.

29. Cavo M, Terpos E, Nanni C, et al. Role of ^{18}F-FDG PET/CT in the diagnosis and management of multiple myeloma and other plasma cell disorders: a consensus statement by the International Myeloma Working Group. Lancet Oncol 2017;18:e206–17.

30. Zamagni E, Nanni C, Patriarca F, et al. A prospective comparison of ^{18}F-fluorodeoxyglucose positron emission tomography-computed tomography, magnetic resonance imaging and whole-body planar radiographs in the assessment of bone disease in newly diagnosed multiple myeloma. Haematologica 2007;92:50–5.

31. Shortt CP, Gleeson TG, Breen KA, et al. Whole-body MRI versus PET in assessment of multiple myeloma disease activity. AJR Am J Roentgenol 2009;192: 980–6.

32. Derlin T, Peldschus K, Münster S, et al. Comparative diagnostic performance of ^{18}F-FDG PET/CT versus whole-body MRI for determination of remission status in multiple myeloma after stem cell transplantation. Eur Radiol 2013;23:570–8.

33. Bartel TB, Haessler J, Brown TL, et al. ^{18}F-fluorodeoxyglucose positron emission tomography in the context of other imaging techniques and prognostic factors in multiple myeloma. Blood 2009;114:2068–76.

34. Durie BG, Kyle RA, Belch A, et al, Scientific Advisors of the International Myeloma Foundation. Myeloma management guidelines: a consensus report from the Scientific Advisors of the International Myeloma Foundation. Hematol J 2003;4(6):379–98.

35. Siontis B, Kumar S, Dispenzieri A, et al. Positron emission tomography-computed tomography in the diagnostic evaluation of smoldering multiple myeloma: identification of patients needing therapy. Blood Cancer J 2015;5:e364.

36. Zamagni E, Nanni C, Gay F, et al. 18F-FDG PET/CT focal, but not osteolytic, lesions predict the progression of smoldering myeloma to active disease. Leukemia 2016;30:417–22.

37. Moulopoulos LA, Dimopoulos MA, Weber D, et al. Magnetic resonance imaging in the staging of solitary plasmacytoma of bone. J Clin Oncol 1993;11: 1311–5.

38. Liebross RH, Ha CS, Cox JD, et al. Solitary bone plasmacytoma: outcome and prognostic factors following radiotherapy. Int J Radiat Oncol Biol Phys 1998;41:1063–7.

39. Lu YY, Chen JH, Lin WY, et al. FDG PET or PET/CT for detecting intramedullary and extramedullary lesions in multiple Myeloma: a systematic review and meta-analysis. Clin Nucl Med 2012;37:833–7.

40. Usmani SZ, Heuck C, Mitchell A, et al. Extramedullary disease portends poor prognosis in multiple myeloma and is over-represented in high-risk disease even in the era of novel agents. Haematologica 2012;97:1761–7.

41. Usmani SZ, Mitchell A, Waheed S, et al. Prognostic implications of serial 18-fluoro-deoxyglucose emission tomography in multiple myeloma treated with total therapy 3. Blood 2013;121(10):1819–23.

42. Lapa C, Lückerath K, Malzahn U, et al. 18 FDG-PET/CT for prognostic stratification of patients with multiple myeloma relapse after stem cell transplantation. Oncotarget 2014;5:7381–91.

43. Derlin T, Weber C, Habermann CR, et al. 18F-FDG PET/CT for detection and localization of residual or recurrent disease in patients with multiple myeloma after stem cell transplantation. Eur J Nucl Med Mol Imaging 2012;39:493–500.

44. Moreau P, Attal M, Karlin L, et al. Prospective evaluation of MRI and PET-CT at diagnosis and before maintenance therapy in symptomatic patients with multiple myeloma included in the IFM/DFCI 2009 trial. Blood 2015;126:395.

45. Beksac M, Gunduz M, Ozen M, et al. Impact of PET-CT response on survival parameters following autologous stem cell transplantation among patients with multiple myeloma: comparison of two cut-off values. Blood 2014;124:3983.

46. Spinnato P, Bazzocchi A, Brioli A, et al. Contrast enhanced MRI and ^{18}F-FDG PET-CT in the assessment of multiple myeloma: a comparison of results in different phases of the disease. Eur J Radiol 2012;81:4013–8.

47. Rubini G, Niccoli-Asabella A, Ferrari C, et al. Myeloma bone and extra-medullary disease: role of PET/CT and other whole-body imaging techniques. Crit Rev Oncol Hematol 2016;101:169–83.

Printed and bound by CPI Group (UK) Ltd, Croydon, CR0 4YY

03/10/2024

01040370-0010